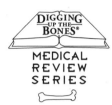

Psychiatry

Notice

Medicine is an ever-changing science. As new research and clinical experience broaden our knowledge, changes in treatment and drug therapy are required. The authors and publisher of this work have checked with sources believed to be reliable in their efforts to provide information that is complete and generally in accord with the standards accepted at the time of publication. However, in view of the possibility of human error or changes in medical sciences, neither the authors nor the publisher nor any other party who has been involved in the preparation or publication of this work warrants that the information contained herein is in every respect accurate or complete, and they are not responsible for any errors or omissions or for the results obtained from use of such information. Readers are encouraged to confirm the information contained herein with other sources. For example and in particular, readers are advised to check the product information sheet included in the package of each drug they plan to administer to be certain that the information contained in this book is accurate and that changes have not been made in the recommended dose or in the contraindications for administration. This recommendation is of particular importance in connection with new or infrequently used drugs.

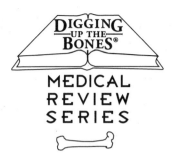

Psychiatry

Compiled and Written by
Nikos M. Linardakis, M.D.

McGraw-Hill
Health Professions Division

New York St. Louis San Francisco Auckland Bogotá Caracas Lisbon London
Madrid Mexico City Milan Montreal New Delhi San Juan Singapore Sydney
Tokyo Toronto

McGraw-Hill

A Division of The McGraw-Hill Companies

PSYCHIATRY: Digging Up the Bones

Copyright © 1998 by *The McGraw-Hill Companies, Inc.* All rights reserved. Printed in the United States of America. Except as permitted under the United States Copyright Act of 1976, no part of this publication may be reproduced or distributed in any form or by any means, or stored in a data base or retrieval system, without prior written permission of the publisher.

1234567890 MALMAL 998

ISBN 0-07-038219-0

This book was set in Times Roman.

Malloy Lithographing, Inc., was the printer and binder.

Cataloging-in-Publication Data is on file for this title at the Library of Congress.

To my mother Lambrini Linardakis

In memory of my father, Michalis J. Linardakis, M.D., for his endless generosity to medicine and psychiatry.

Contents

Preface ix
Acknowledgments xi

Chapter 1
General Psychiatry Highlights 7

Chapter 2
Disorders of Infancy, Childhood or Adolescence 17

Chapter 3
Delirium, Dementia, & Cognitive Disorders 25

Chapter 4
Mental Disorders secondary to Medical Conditions 29

Chapter 5
Disorders secondary to Substances 31

Chapter 6
Schizophrenia & Psychotic Disorders 39

Chapter 7
Mood Disorders 47

Chapter 8
Anxiety Disorders 53

Chapter 9
Somatoform & Factitious Disorders 57

Chapter 10
Dissociative Disorders 59

Chapter 11
Sexual & Gender Identity Disorders 61

Chapter 12
Eating Disorders 63

Chapter 13
Sleep Disorders 65

Chapter 14
Adjustment & Personality Disorders 67

Chapter 15
Neuropsychiatry Highlights 71

Chapter 16
Psychopharmacology & Other Treatments 99

Index   109

Preface

The sixth volume of the *Digging Up the Bones* medical review series was created to present the clinical portion of medical training, psychiatry. We begin the review as an introduction to the psychiatric examination and then into the areas of psychiatry, including disorders, substance abuse, personality disorders, sexual disorders, eating disorders, psychopharmacology, neuropsychiatry, and other aspects of psychiatry. Please take the time to understand all of the concepts presented.

The contents of *Digging Up the Bones* medical review series *Psychiatry* has been arranged in an order established in consideration of *DSM-IV*. This was created to present material in a sequence similar to that found in the classification manual, and thus aid in the learning or use of the *DSM-IV* manual in the future.

It is appropriate to note that this review series was created as a concise *summary* of the different diagnoses, treatments, and related facts within medicine. In this volume of psychiatry, we will cover most topics that are heavily tested on examinations such as the USMLE and course examinations. We know you will appreciate its *brief* and *concise* presentation of the facts within psychiatry that will increase your mastery of this necessary material to help in your general medicine practice in the future. For simplification, I may refer to the physician/student/caretaker, who is interviewing a patient, as the "examiner."

Digging Up the Bones medical review series has received recognition from around the world through the shared comments with physicians and students. Your mastery of these psychiatry facts should improve your clinical skills. I know your efforts will pay off, and you will share these skills with others in the years to come.

Now, let's get started!

Nikos M. Linardakis, M.D.

Acknowledgments

Many appreciative thank you's to several of my colleagues. An enormous appreciation to Alexander Z. Golbin, M.D., Ph. D., for his influence and guidance in the formation of this volume of *Digging Up the Bones* in psychiatry. His contributions to this work promises a second edition in the near future with his added assistance.

My gratitude to my friend and all-time "little sister," Melissa Klimala. Her help in the original manuscript, typing and editing, greatly assisted in the completion of the book.

I admire the generous input and encouragement of my friends and colleagues at the Chicago Medical School, University of Illinois School of Medicine, Northwestern University Medical School, University of Utah School of Medicine, Iowa Osteopathic Medical School, University of California Medical Schools and several other medical schools.

I wish to thank the several students and physicians who encouraged me in the completion of this book, including, Michael Chen, M.D., William Magdalin, M.D., Sonia Lott, Timothy McCarthy, several students who have written to the publisher, and to the several American Medical Student Association class presidents I visited with at the annual meetings in the past few years. A special thank you to Janna Blake for the informative news release prior to publication. Your valuable comments and contributions represented key concepts and the added support leading to the creation of this and other volumes in the *Digging Up the Bones* medical review series.

1
General Psychiatry Highlights

Examination
During an examination of a patient:
Interact with the patient by conversing. Ask questions and observe the patient's behavior and reactions. Remember, begin the evaluation as soon as you first see the patient. (i.e., the initial greeting, when entering the room, or other). Create trust and compliance with the patient by setting a good tone in the interview. Do not immediately discuss medical problems or a "cold" review of the patient's problems. The doctor should take extra steps in making the individual comfortable: do not have a desk between the patient, (instead, position seats kiddie corner to each other, this will decrease the anxiety), be relaxed, if you are nervous looking, imagine the patient. Also, be serious with terminology, your patient is intelligent and may be much more than yourself. Use humor tastefully, if the patient is trying to be humorous (even if it is a delusion), feel free to laugh or join in. All of the above are involved in the evaluation for the diagnosis, it may also contribute to the therapy. This evaluation can be considered a *process* to diagnose patients. Included in this process are: clinical presentation, behavior, history, lab results. This is all directed to diagnose and begin a proper treatment plan.

DSM-IV™ (Diagnostic and Statistical Manual-Fourth Edition)
DSM-IV™ is the manual in psychiatry that follows criteria to determine the diagnosis. It is the "gold-standard" book of psychiatry, but is often not used properly. This is an important book to understand, since it sets the criteria for proper diagnosis of the psychiatric patient. Diagnosis is then decided by a process of exclusion or inclusion. It increases the probability of a correct diagnosis by associating signs and symptoms. The form of organization is called the *Multiaxial System* and includes:
    Axis I: Clinical Disorders, Other Conditions that may be a focus of clinical attention.
    Axis II: Personality Disorders, Mental Retardation
    Axis III: General Medical Conditions
    Axis IV: Psychosocial BL Environmental Problems
    Axis V: Global Assessment of Functioning

Making the Diagnosis

Look for Characteristics	Associated with:
Hallucinations	Schizophrenia
Delusions	Mood Disorders

Depressive features
  Sad Mood
  Lack of motivation,
  Loss of interest
	Depression

Guilt, Early wakening	Melancholia
Irritable mood, hyperactivity rapid/pressured speech	Mania Bipolar affective disorder (Manic-Depressive)
Altered consciousness (changed level of arousal) Rambling speech, Agitation, Cognitive impairment	Delirium
Clear consciousness Diffuse cognitive impairment	Dementia
Slurred speech, Breath odor = alcohol	Alcohol Intoxication
Anxiety, Obsessive-compulsive	Systemic illness
Dementia with ataxia and urinary incontinence	Normal-pressure hydrocephaly

Knowing the available choices, observing behavior, and reviewing laboratory results will help in determining the diagnosis. Treatment begins after proper evaluation and diagnosis (you want to avoid administering "therapeutic" medication that may not be "treating" the *real* problem). Don't rush the diagnosis that may result in the wrong treatment. This will decrease iatrogenic morbidity like tardive dyskinesia from improper medication).

Recognize signs, symptoms, and behavior of the individual *subjectively*. Then, *objectively* observe the patient and obtain lab values.

Use precise terms to identify the behavior. Understand the difference between the *form*, and the *content* of material (i.e., a hallucinated voice). For example, what and when the voice occurs, if it is clear and how long it lasts. Was there any precipitating event to bring the "voice" on? Was there any other hallucination before or after the event (i.e., a strange taste)? The *form* of psychiatric illness is similar across cultures, just the *content* changes.

Melancholic patients have the same *form* (sadness, insomnia, and guilty feelings) as depression, but the *content* of their guilty ideas is different (melancholic patients do not anticipate killing themselves; they feel really down).

In making a diagnosis in psychiatry, the examiner must make decisions for treatment based on the patient's behavior, examination and laboratory assessment.

For example, if there is deviant behavior, is it a pathological illness or is it a personality disorder or social problem? Will the treatment begin with medications or psychosocial therapy (behavior modification)?

First, determine the patient's chief complaint. Decide the problems that can create this "chief complaint". Create a differential list (differential diagnosis) of: a psychiatric or personality disorder, social problems, and metabolic diseases or thyroid disease, etc.

The DSM-IV™ manual gives the latest official list of the different choices for the differential. Categories will include: affective disorders, anxiety disorders, and others (we will review the majority of disorders in this book). The International Classification of Diseases, 9th Ed. (ICD-9) shows the other choices, like: CNS diseases and other systemic diseases. Those patients that do not meet the criteria for any diagnosis, are placed in the "Not Otherwise Specified" (NOS) category.

Problems with Speech and Language
Language disorders: When verbal communication lacks logical organization and is difficult to understand. Abnormal speech from abnormal thinking. This thought disorder can appear in: the expressed speech, the content, the gestures and other forms of speech coherence.

Formal thought disorder is similar to aphasia. Thought disorders propose that there are other disorders present. In acute coarse brain disorders (like intoxication) look for: rambling speech, and in chronic disorders like dementia or mania): flight of ideas, non-sequiturs, driveling speech, perseveration, derailment, and tangential speech.

Speech and language *form* differs from thought *content*. The speech *form* depends on the rate and rhythm, the grammar, and syntax (or sentence formation). *Form* is *how* a patient speaks, NOT *what* he is speaking about. This is the *content* or *what* is being spoken about, and is of less value when diagnosing a patient. Use common sense in recognizing the content of speech: realize that it IS important to recognize depressive thoughts, hopelessness and other expressions seen with other illnesses.

Forms of speech	Characteristic of:
Hesitant speech	Huntington's chorea
Slow or hesitant speech	Depression, Altered consciousness, Coarse brain disorders.
Rapid and pressured speech	Mania, Anxiety.
Coprolalia (unrestrained profanity)	Gilles de Tourette's Syndrome
Scanning ("stretched") speech	Multiple sclerosis
Staccato ("chopped") speech	Partial Epilepsy
Adult onset stuttering	Extrapyramidal lesions

Psychopathology
Expression of deviant brain structure or function. Neurologic disease or *organic mental disorders*. Interaction and care for the patient begins with a neuropsychiatric evaluation: detailed history, systemic, neurologic, and mental status examination. This may also include necessary laboratory tests. A final diagnosis is made and a proper treatment is prescribed.

Women have a higher risk than men for affective and some anxiety disorders. Anxiety disorder develops earlier in life; whereas, bipolar affective disorder develops during the third decade of life.

Thought Disorder	Findings
Speech of Aphasic patients	Jargon speech, Driveling speech
Circumlocutory speech	Calling something by its *function or other characteristics*, rather than by its name. (i.e., a watch becomes "the thing that tells the time.") Not precise; vague.
Word approximation	Saying "writer," for a pen or pencil; describes the meaning of the word, but **not** the *exact* name.
Out-of-class semantic or Paraphasia	Utterance that has no meaning to others. A made-up word.
Tangential speech	Inability to finish the logical goal of the speech. (After the person continues on and on, you find yourself asking "What is the point?")

Abnormal speech can be present with schizophrenia, aphasia, mania, etc.

First, evaluate the patient's **appearance**:

Appearance	Possible Disorder
Skinny person with low fat : muscle ratio (**ecto**morph)	Schizophrenia
Large, heavy person with high fat : muscle ratio (**endo**morph)	Affective disorder
A tattooed person	An antisocial personality
A dazed, ataxic woman *urinated*	Normal-Pressure Hydrocephalus

Appearance (**body form**) related to Psychiatric Condition:

Body Feature	Associated With
Endomorph	Affective disorder, Bipolar Affective disorder (Manic depressive)
Ectomorph	Schizophrenia

Next, look at the **motor behavior**:
Describe the patient's gait, if there are any abnormal movements, or coordination problems (motor disturbances).

Types motor behavior	Associated with:
Motor retardation	Depression
Head-rubbing	Schizophrenia
Wide-based or ataxic gait	An alcoholic
Hesitant gait	Huntington's chorea
"Shuffling" gait	Frontal lobe disease
Picking at bed sheets	Delirium
bouncing and tiptoe gaits ("scuttling" gait)	Catatonia
Agitation (a motor disturbance)	Psychotic behavior
Shifting body positions, playing with fingers	Anxiety

Agitation
Increased motor behavior without any particular goal (i.e., continuously moving around). This is the *motor* expression of increased arousal or mood, that appears as: Anxiety, Anger, or Sadness.

Psychosis
Psychotic patients have socially deviant behavior, which includes talking to themselves or shouting to the air.

Tardive dyskinesia
Results from *chronic* ingestion of *neuroleptics*. These patients have continuous jerky fine movements. Also, feet tapping and repetitive oral movements (i.e., lip smacking or in-and-out movements of the tongue). These movements may worsen with a stressful event.

*Hyper*activity
Patient doing many things at one time, or having many conversations. Cardiovascular collapse and sometimes death may occur with those very excited patients who do not receive therapy. This type of excessive hyperactivity is seen in patients who have *mania*.

*Hypo*activity
A non-reacting patient, who does not move for a long time. *Excessive* hypoactivity is called **stupor**. These patients are motionless for hours, stare, or are mute and unresponsive. This is also the response to painful stimuli. It is considered **akinetic mutism syndrome** when there is stupor with coarse brain disease.

Mannerisms Strange movements like: hopping instead of walking, saluting people and any exaggerated movements.

Automatic obedience
Even though the patient is told *not* to copy what the examiner is doing, the patient does it anyway. (This is also seen in catatonic patients.)

Motor behavior is regulated by the *frontal* lobe. Therefore, motor problems (i.e., hyperactivity) are associated with brain disease in this area. *Drug-induced* abnormal movements are similar to *spontaneous* abnormal movements. Irregular *spontaneous* movements include: grimacing, ballistic arm and hand movements, hyperkinesis (increased motor activity), and other behaviors.

Drug-induced abnormal movements
(We must remember that all psychotherapeutic drugs affect motor function.)

Drug	Associated with/causes
Tri-cyclic antidepressants	Irritability
Lithium	Persistent, fine tremors
	Coordination problems with impaired fine motor movements
	With long-term treatment or toxicity: Coarse tremors Ataxia Myoclonus
Monoamine oxidase inhibitors	Agitation
Anxiolytics	With increased doses may induce: Ataxia, tremors, and myoclonus.
Neuroleptics (Phenothiazines)	Altered motor behavior Potent inducer of extrapyramidal signs. Parkinsonism; bradykinesia and tremor

Neuroleptics
Features of drug-induced parkinsonism: expressionless face, slow motor activity, a "stiff" appearance, and micrographia (real *tiny writing*). Many patients on neuroleptics may show this parkinsonism, especially women and very young and very old patients. The following can be seen with neuroleptic treatment.

Dystonias
Spontaneous muscle spasms that occur in the first days of treatment with neuroleptics. These will have cramps and spasms of the muscles (usually in the facial area). Dystonias also increase with the more potent drugs.

Akathesia
Motor restlessness. Basically, the patient cannot stand still. This happens in 1 of 5 patients after a couple of weeks on neuroleptic medication, occurring more in the first months of treatment.

Neuroleptics (continued)

Dyskinesias
Difficulty with performing voluntary movements, abnormal motility, and involuntary movements (like tardive *dyskinesia*). Tongue protrusion, lip smacking, and shoulder shrugging.

Tardive dyskinesia (TD)
Many abnormal movements from long-term treatment with neuroleptics (see below for list of symptoms). Following months of treatment, tardive dyskinesia may appear after decreasing or stopping neuroleptic treatment. As much as 1 of 2 patients on long-term therapy may develop this problem, especially the elderly. T.D. is apparently IRreversible!!! The examiner must rate the motor abnormalities using a rating scale. Some of the characteristic symptoms (which worsen with stress) include:
  (Choreiform movements of the buccal-lingual-fascial muscles.)
  Irregular movements of the tongue (protrusion and curling) and cheeks,
  Gait and postural movements,
  Choreo-athetoid movements of the extremities,
  Ballistic arm movements, shifting of weight, lordosis, rocking and swaying, pelvic thrusting, and vocalizations and dysphagias.

Mood
Mood is the *emotion* of the person at a particular time. An altered mood is associated with most psychiatric illnesses. Being upset, sad, happy, angry or anxious. The mood establishes a person's behavior and can change the heart rate, blood pressure, and other physiological responses. Furthermore, a change in mood will affect speech, thought, and may develop delusional thoughts. To understand the difference between mood and affect, let us first realize that *mood* is considered the *content* of affect. And, *affect* is the *expression* of the mood; or, *affect* is the *behavior* resulting from the mood.

Affect
Again, affect is the *expression* of the mood. In other words, affect is the *behavior* that *expresses* the mood. Affect has an intensity, a range, and stability. Affect also has appropriateness and quality of mood, and relatedness. Here are two examples: affective disorder patients may have a *constant* mood of irritability. Schizophrenics show *no* mood and appear emotionally blunted.

Affect (continued)

> **Range** of affect = change in expression of emotions over time (i.e., a constant mood or one mood = "constricted" range of affect). This could be seen in a depressed patient expressing only sadness and therefore has a *constricted* affect. And in those who have rapid mood changes (one moment they are very happy, then angry, then crying). This is called a *labile* affect or unstable emotions.
>
> **Intensity** of affect = the degree of emotional expression (i.e., the degree of arousal). Rage > anger, and euphoria > happiness.
>
> **Appropriateness** = if the patient's mood expression and behavior is normal or abnormal for a situation. Inappropriateness of mood occurs in illnesses, but can occur in a situation which may show anxiety and not a real pathology (i.e., when a person laughs when something went terribly wrong). Such behaviors are used in the diagnosis of a patient.
>
> **Relatedness** = the ability of a person to express and interact with others. Loss of relatedness is seen in dementia and in schizophrenia. There is a deterioration of personality and changes in the person's behavior and interests. Emotional blunting = *loss of* emotional expression.
>
> *Emotional expression* is evaluated by the *facial expressions*, tone of voice, speech and gestures; notice the mood and the range of affect. *Loss of* emotional expression = motor *aprosodia*, usually from neurologic problems of the *non*dominant frontal region of the brain (motor aphasia occurs with problems in the *dominant* frontal area).
>
> Aprosodia present with a *loss of*: facial expression, emotions, gestures, and mood. Also the patient has a monotonous voice and difficulty in expressing any feelings. Neurologically, frontal cortical atrophy is found.
>
> **Volition** deals with planning, motivation, and desires. The worst form of *loss of* volition is seen with the lack of personal hygiene and grooming. These patients can**not** *plan for the future*. This is seen in patients with schizophrenia; there is apathy and unrelatedness, and a decreased intensity of mood. They show limited affection and show little concern. Usually they have no friends.

2
Disorders of Infancy, Childhood or Adolescence

Child Development

Biological (genetics) and *environmental* influences (family interaction, social, cultural, and stressful events) affect human development. Areas of development include: gross and fine motor, speech, cognition, perception, social, and emotional development. Children may develop at very different rates. After a clinical observation, the examiner may assess the child's *developmental milestones*, cognitive and social development by administering the Denver Developmental Screening Test, the Gesell Infant Scale, the Wechsler Intelligence Scale for Children-Revised, and other behavioral scales.

Approx. Age	**Developmental Milestones (Behavior)**
0 - 6 months	Innate motor reflexes, perception of stimulation Crying and looking at faces of others is form of emotional, social, and communication level.
6 months up to one year old	Stability develops, (*gross* movements: sitting upright, rolls over; and *fine* movements: moving and touching things with more coordination) Crying, laughing, babbling, and *stranger* anxiety.
1 year old	Movement develops, (*gross* movements: walking; and *fine* movements: controlling different objects) Uses words, anger, and other emotions. *Separation* anxiety.
1 1/2 years (18 months)	Interacting. (*gross* movements: climbing; and fine movements: coordinating and using different objects) Increasing vocabulary to almost 100 words. Very emotional.
2 years old	Environmental. (*gross* movements: running; and *fine* movements: copies a circle)
3 years old	Planning. (*gross* movements: jumping; and *fine* movements: copies a cross)

Sigmund Freud and the Psychoanalytic Theory

Freud described three systems of the mind: the unconscious, preconscious, and conscious. First, the *unconscious* develops (this is the irrational, wishful thinking part). Later, as the child controls his actions by becoming more rational, the *conscious* system develops. These related areas of the mind were also discussed as the id, the ego, and the superego. The **id** is mainly instinct and fulfills pleasure and wishes, with no concept of reality. The **ego** develops after the mind matures and deals with reality. Finally, the **superego** is the person's conscience, and is related to the role models usually given by the ethics of the parents. These three parts interact and form the personality of the person as he gets older.

Freud also discussed the development of the child in stages based on genetics and age. (*For additional discussion of these stages please review* <u>Digging Up the Bones</u>...® <u>Volume 5: Behavioral Science</u>) The stages and the associated development include:
   the oral phase (dependence or aggression),
   the anal phase (possessive and organized),
   the phallic phase ("Oedipus complex", and same-sex parent relation; conscience),
   latency (skills formation)
   adolescence (sexual development and peer interest).

A child develops behavior continuously, and therefore it is difficult to designate a simple pathological behavior as in adults. Illnesses in psychiatry appear with various signs and symptoms at different times of development. Treatment may aid or hinder the development of the child, be careful of the management you choose.

Furthermore, *environment* influences the growing *child* more than an adult. You can easily see the effects of family, school, or church on a growing child. From a "problem" family, can arise a "problem" child. Pathological findings in a family tend to appear in the individual child. School can also influence a child's development (especially at 5-6 years old). The parents, siblings, teachers, and others should recognize changes or abnormalities. The child is more sensitive, and the family should not "label" the child as "abnormal" or having a disability (this will create a problem for the child). Adult psychiatric diagnoses are often seen in children, although the diagnostic criteria are different.

Adult Diagnoses	Childhood Signs/Symptoms
Major Depressive Disorder *Depressed* mood	*Irritable* mood
PTSD Recurrent thoughts of fear	Uneasy and disordered

Developmental Disorders

Psychopathology <---can create---> delay. Examples include: mental retardation, sensory problems, problems with socialization, lack of self-esteem, poor motor and speech skills, communication problems, and emotional and cognitive dysfunction. Delays in development is a serious problem which may lead to deficits in motor, social and language skills. *Chronological* age and *developmental* age differences may signal a problem with development. Patient may not be able to perform the skills of an individual with the same chronological age. A delay in reaching milestones, irregular behavior, and decreased self-esteem will result. Physical problems also are related with developmental delay. The causes of developmental delay include: metabolic errors of the newborn, toxins (like lead poisoning), and genetic abnormalities.

Learning Disorders (LD)

Delayed development of motor, language or cognitive skills (especially when compared to IQ). Learning disorders occur in children who have *learning* problems and this does not correlate with their *intellectual* ability (normal to high I.Q.). Special education classes and learning techniques can improve learning, decrease school failure, and improve self-esteem. Disorders include: reading (dyslexia), mathematics and written expression. Associated conditions: lead poisoning, fetal alcohol syndrome, conduct disorder, and attention deficit hyperactivity disorder. LD's are found in approximately 5% of children, failure to diagnose may result in poor self-esteem, and interfere in school and occupation. Unknown etiology, may be a CNS problem from genetic or environmental insults.

Mental Retardation

Poorly, delayed cognitive skills and an I.Q. (intelligence quotient) that is below average (<70). These children have social difficulties. Diagnosis is usually made by the age of 5-6 years old (school time). Majority of mentally retarded individuals are *mildly* retarded (NOT severely retarded). Usually severely retarded individuals have more associated *medical* conditions like: metabolic, endocrine, physical, neurological, genito-urinary, and genetic problems. It is common to have problems with lack of self-esteem and to be impulsive. Consider in the differential diagnosis of mental retardation: learning disorders, sensory problems, sensory deprivation from lack of maternal care. Prevalence = 1 %.

Associations	Etiology (Results from):
Mild mental retardation	Idiopathic
Genetic abnormalities (Chromosome)	Metabolic error: Glycogen storage dis. lipidoses, Chromosomal: Down's Syndrome (Trisomy 21), Cri du Chat (chr. 5).
Acquired	Viral: Herpes, CMV Bacterial: GBS (group B strep) Toxins: lead or heavy metals Environmental: Deprived social/family care

Mildly retarded individuals can acquire a fifth to sixth grade academic level. Several social problems are apparent; including: impulse problems, and lack of self-esteem. They can function on their own.

Moderately retarded individuals are at a second grade level, and perform daily duties. Social problems create difficulties for these individuals. Some Down's Syndrome patients are moderately impaired, but function fairly well in everyday life.

Severely retarded individuals are usually a result of poisonings, lack of prenatal care, physical trauma, and infections (i.e., viral or group B strep intrauterine infection). More males then females.

Treatment should be directed to *prenatal care and genetic counseling* for prevention of retardation. Then, mothers over 35 years old or in high risk pregnancy may have a paracentesis to check for chromosomal abnormalities. Academic evaluation and appropriate accommodation or special education classes should be provided early on. The environment can effect the esteem and social function of the individual; "Special Olympics", summer camps, and other support groups and events create increased awareness and support for the development of these individuals. Retardation could effect every member of a family, proper behavioral guidance can create a heart-warming and caring family.

Attention Deficit Hyperactivity Disorder (ADHD)
ADHD used to be called "minimal brain dysfunction". The behavior of the child includes: Aggressive, irritable, lack of attention, poor in school. Chronic impairment since childhood. The problem of "not being able to sit still, always on the go", the person is continuously getting into fights, and dose poorly in school because of the inattention. There is inattention and hyperactivity with impulsive behavior lasting at least 6 months and occurring before the age of 7. These children develop poor self-esteem and have behavioral problems due to the continuous "don't do that!" response from parents and peers. They require special learning techniques in school because of their lack of attention and easy distractibility. ADHD is often seen in relatives. Treatment is with amphetamines (Ritalin® or Methvlphenidate; Cylert® or pemoline; Dexedrine® or dextroamphetamine), behavioral techniques, and improved learning techniques. Treatment does NOT show potential adult drug abuse. Many ADHD patients have additional learning disabilities that are exacerbated with the ADHD.

Autistic Disorder
The person lacks the social interaction and has impaired communication. Intrauterine *rubella* can cause autistic disorder, but it is most likely due to problems in the development of the CNS. Other medical conditions include: encephalitis, phenylketonuria, tuberous sclerosis, Fragile X syndrome, and anoxia or from unknown etiology. Associated with: mental retardation, motor behaviors, emotional problems, hearing impairment, and self-injurious behavior. Autism has an early onset (by 3 years of age), and has impaired communication with irregular or absent speech, with repetitive stereotyped behavior. The patient is preoccupied with repetitive motor movements that have no purpose. Injurious behavior like biting, head banging, and body rocking may occur. Abnormalities may be seen in EEG and there is a male to female predominance (5 males: 1 female). Increased serotonin has been suggested. The movie, *Rain Man*, portrayed an adult with Autistic Disorder who had several motor repetitive activities, and mannerisms with other disabilities.

Conduct Disorder
"Juvenile delinquents"; These individuals disrupt society with aggressive behavior, theft and deceit, vandalism, and going against rules. They go against social norms. Conduct disorder persons are: fire-setters, robbers, liars, vandals, run-aways...It starts before 10 years old or during adolescence, with a familial pattern like ADHD and anti-social personality disorder. Treatment includes: build a moral responsibility in the individual, teaching right from wrong, build a positive social identity.

Oppositional Defiant Disorder
Similar to conduct disorder. But, these individuals only defy authority persons. They are very temperamental and negative, causing problems with authorities and adults. The *parents* are a possible *cause* of the problem and therefore a "treatment" is educating parents on child rearing.

Social Phobia
Previously called Avoidant Disorder of childhood. Social phobia is characterized by: normal interaction with known persons, but incredible shyness to strangers. Treatment includes: behavioral techniques with assertion training.

Pervasive Developmental Disorders
These include Autistic Disorder, Asperger's Disorder, Rett's Disorder

Eating Disorders of Childhood
These include:
PICA
Having an appetite for "food" that is unfit for consumption; like wanting to eat wood or coal (nonnutritive substances).

Rumination disorder
Regurgitation and rechewing food (yes, like how animals ruminate). This lasts for at least 1 month, and there is NO other medical problem (like reflux).

Tic Disorders
Involuntary movements or vocalizations like: Tourette's Disorder (uncontrolled vocalization of foul language), and Tic Disorders.

Gilles de la Tourette's (GTS)
Tourette's Syndrome is a disorder of vocal and motor tics, coprolalia (sudden foul language; i.e., "sh_t" repeated quickly), and echolalia. Usually seen in Whites (Not in African-Americans), and Males. Starts as a child up until about 16 years old. In this disorder we find characteristics like: *tics, repetitive movements, echolalia* and *echopraxia*. **Tics** occur with: the *eyes, vocalizations* (pathologic coughing, barking, throat clearing; making irregular sounds), and coprolalia (uncontrolled swearing). **Repetitive movements** include: hitting, touching, and stamping feet. It is also associated with self-injurious behavior and sleep disorders. Familial, and usually seen in males. GTS has compulsions, and family history of tics. Both have an early age of onset, lifetime symptoms come and go, these are unwanted behaviors, and therefore is similar to Obsessive-Compulsive Disorder. The treatment includes: *Haloperidol* or *Clomipramine (Anafranil)*, and behavioral therapy.

Childhood Anxiety
Anxiety disorders are unrealistic fears or anxiousness that is at an inappropriate level. Symptoms include: physical problems "stomach ache" fears of the "boogy man" and other phobias, sleeping irregularities, and nail biting.
Stranger anxiety is the fear of strangers (occurs from **8 months** to 2 years). *Separation* anxiety is the fear of separation from the parent (occurs from **1 year** to 3 years old). Separation anxiety *disorder* is associated with stress as a loss of a relative or other illness. It appears as an increased anxiety from being separated from a care-giver or other attached person or pet. It is more common in females and appears in somatic complaints. Treatment includes: changing family routines, benzodiazepines, and behavioral techniques like systematic desensitization.
Phobia is a fear that is not logical (occurs from 3 to 6 years).

Generalized Anxiety Disorder in childhood
Was called Overanxious disorder of childhood. The child is unrealistically anxious and worries about...everything! "What will happen, what happened, am I good enough?" Increased incidence in the first born child, upper socio-economic group and achievers. The perfectionists, with self-doubt and somatic complaints, habits and phobias. They avoid performance activities and can develop into social phobia in adulthood. Treatment: teaching the child that they don't need to please, and accepting failure; Benzodiazepines may improve response.

Elimination disorders
Very common, Enuresis (or abnormal urination), and Encopresis (or inappropriate defecation) that is NOT due to a medical condition or the physiologic effect of a substance.
Enuresis
Repeated urination in bed or in the child's pants. It is done with intention or involuntarily. 2 times/week for at least 3 months, or having social or academic problems. The child has to be at least at a developmental age to control urination (5 years old).

Encopresis
Repeated feces in inappropriate locations, like on the floor! It has to occur at a developmental level (4 years old), and it is done with intention or **in**voluntarily.

Pervasive Developmental Disorders
Autistic Disorder
The impaired social interaction, with stereotyped and repetitive behavior or language. Stereotyped motor mannerisms include: hand flapping and other irregular repetitive movements.

Rett's Disorder
Normal development in the first 5 months of life, then there is a loss of skills and a decrease in head growth. The child has poor coordination, and has psychomotor retardation. (Social interaction will develop later.)

Asperger's Disorder
Impaired social interaction, includes problems with: eye gaze, expressions of the face, and social development. Repetitive and stereotyped behaviors are also present. These children have problems in social and working environments.

3
Delirium, Dementia, & Cognitive Disorders

Delirium and Dementia
Both have cognitive problems. But, Delirium is an altered level of consciousness and usually is an *acute* problem. Dementia usually is *chronic*.

Delirium
Altered consciousness <u>and</u> impaired cognitive function. Patient is disoriented, lacks attention, and has several problems with memory and processing. Possible medical problem or drug abuse/intoxication as the etiology. On lab exam see: electrolyte imbalance, abnormal liver or thyroid function tests, EEG abnormalities, and findings in toxicology. May be due to infection, liver or renal dysfunction, inappropriate drug levels or head trauma.

Dementia
Impaired cognitive function and memory problems. May be caused by long-term substance abuse, and other medical problems. The person has mental deterioration, and emotional lability (happy one minute, then sad the next). Problems with development as a child. Seen in 1 of 5 elderly individuals, and may have sudden or gradual onset. Heritable dementia: Alzheimer's Disease, Huntington's disease. May be due to: CNS infection, trauma, hydrocephalus, and vitamin B12 deficiency. Treatment includes recognizing a causative agent and social support. (see below for different types of dementia and related findings)

Amnestic Disorder
Impaired memory (but, with clear consciousness and cognition). This usually occurs suddenly. Due to: damage to the hippocampus (causing a problem with memory), or drug-induced. This is seen with thiamine deficiency in alcoholics and the loss of memory.

Delirium
Again, it is an acute cognitive impairment with altered consciousness. Caused by: trauma to the head (accident victim), drug and alcohol toxicities, infectious or metabolic disease. You want to prevent injury by restraining the patient and decreasing the agitation by giving anxiolytics. Be careful of barbiturates if there is head trauma or other.

Delirium (continued)
Seen with medical illnesses like: hypoglycemia, infection, or fever. Also, renal problems, intoxications, and certain drugs. The person's behavior is disoriented and agitated, with physical problems like: tachycardia, sweating, and cold-clammy skin. On lab exam: the blood glucose may be altered (also, check the blood urea nitrogen, and the electrolytes); check liver function, blood gas, and drug levels. Do an EKG. Go through the causes of delirium. The common ones are drug overdose, epilepsy, head trauma, CNS infection, pulmonary and cardiovascular problems, and other systemic problems like an overwhelming infection.

Overall, look for the signs of delirium, and a change in behavior. Then find the cause of the problem, then treat the patient. Is it due to a drug overdose, or a metabolic problem? If it is due to a low blood sugar level or a lack of oxygen, treat it quickly. Check the patient's blood pressure, the body temperature, and EKG for irregularities.

Dementia
Usually seen in the elderly (5% of persons over 65; and 20% of persons over 80). Risk: African Americans > Euro-Americans. BUT, dementia is NOT a normal aging process. The diffuse cognitive problems appear gradually with memory loss, disorientation, and poor performance on tasks. The patient shows a slow decline in activities and loses interests. Dementia is often mistaken as major depression or other disorder.

Types of Dementias

Alzheimer's Disease
Dementia of the Alzheimer's type (DAT)
First occurs after 50 years old, and usually after 70. This is the most common dementia. Alzheimer's usually presents as: dementia after 65, a decrease in cognitive function, with memory loss. Seen in the majority of first-degree relatives. A familial relationship has been shown with **Down's Syndrome** and **leukemias**. The link is with the Chromosome **21**. Treatment can include: *Tacrine*; increases the Acetylcholine levels within the synaptic cleft.

The overall disease has been categorized into 3 stages. Stage **1** is when the speech and ideas are limited. The person begins to show problems with anemia (inability to name things), dysgraphia (problems writing), some memory problems, and visual-spatial problems. Depression and a loss of interest is seen in this stage.

Types of Dementias

Alzheimer's Disease (continued)

In Stage **2,** there is an increased problem with cognition and behavior. The person sees serious problems with memory, and becomes angry; especially when personal hygiene worsens. In Stage **3** the person has serious deteriorating conditions with incontinence, and the need for continuous care.

Multi-infarct dementia (MID)
The second most common dementia (approximately 10% of dementias). MID occurs around 50 - 60 years old, and is more common in *men* with vascular problems. The infarcts occur due to *hypertension* which causes occluded cerebral vessels, and problems in cognition. Atherosclerosis and other vascular disorders can also cause the MID. Treatment includes: anticoagulants and *aspirin.*

Pick's Disease
Dementia starting *before* 65 years of age, a behavioral change and a decrease in cognitive function, with personality and behavioral changes. The onset is usually between 40 - 60 years old.

Basal Ganglia Disease Dementia
Parkinson's disease
Huntington's disease
Wilson's disease
These are considered **sub**cortical dementias. The person presents with extrapyramidal signs and subcortical problems. Deficits in: psyche-motor, memory, cognitive functions; & mood and speech problems.

White Matter Disease & Dementias
Progressive multifocal encephalopathy, multiple sclerosis, leukodystrophy, AIDS, vitamin deficiency (B12), neurotoxicity, and traumatic brain injury may cause a dementia. The dementia usually develops < 50 years old, with some cognitive problems, but the person has a normal personality.

Treatment of dementia
Some response with treating underlying problems like:
D-penicillamine for Wilson's disease,
Ventricular shunting for NPH (hydrocephalus),
Vitamins for nutritional disorders,
Hormone replacements for endocrine disorders,

Treatment of dementia (continued)
Penicillin for CNS syphilis, and
Surgery for hematomas.
Selegiline (an irreversible MAOI) may help Alzheimer's patients improve in cognitive function; Neuroleptics, Haloperidol for psychosis, ECT for psychotic features with dementia.

Remember, these patients tend to forget things, so the treatment plan requires care-takers because of the lack of self-care, and the problems with personal hygiene. Family and friends should visit often.

4
Mental Disorders secondary to Medical Conditions

Catatonia
Catatonia is identified by hyperactive-hypoactive intervals of motor behavior. When a person is catatonic, he may have an affective disorder or schizophrenia. Diagnosis includes the motor features of mutism and stupor (but, these are *not* pathognomonic). Catatonic symptoms may also be seen after frontal lobe injury (since the frontal lobe is involved in motor control). Catatonia is related with: Irregular gait, extending out a limb (arm) for a long time for no apparent reason, staying in one location for a long time, copying the same movements as another person, repeating speech, prosectic speech = mumbled speech with no volume...these all signal the possibility of *catatonia*.
Treatment: Lorazepam or ECT.

Stupor
Extreme psychomotor inhibition in which the patient doesn't move or speak, and stops eating. Treatment: Initially, *Sodium amobarbital* or a benzodiazepine right before eating, and this helps him have the "energy" to move. ECT is used to treat the patient.

Catatonia
Look for the following on an examination to diagnose catatonia: Stupor, waxy flexibility, catalepsy, mutism, stereotyping, automatic obedience, etc.

> **Stupor** Again, this is extreme *hypo*activity. The person is mute, not moving, and unresponsive to stimuli (even painful stimulation doesn't make the patient respond).

> **Gegen*halt*en** Negativism. Patient *resists* the examiner's force, with the same strength that the examiner applies.

> **Catalepsy** Keeping the same position for long intervals. Positions like: facial and body postures. *Psychologic pillow* is when the patient is in bed with his head lifted to appear as if it is on a pillow. Holding the arms up over the head or in strange positions.

Catatonia (continued)

    Mutism — Inability to respond with speech.

    Waxy flexibility — Resisting movement to a different position, but slowly allowing the change. (Think of molding the *wax* of a candle as it slowly bends as you shape it.)

    Stereotypy — Repetitive movements and behavior or repeated words or phrases (verbal repetition or stereotypy) = *verb*igeration.

    Echolalia — Repetition of what is *said*.

    Echopraxia — Copying *movements* even though the patient is told not to.

Behavioral Changes	Associated with:
Jerky movements	Chronic use of Neuroleptics
Emotional Blunting (Withdrawn and indifferent; lack of emotions.) Problems maintaining school, work, and friendships. (think of the poor street walkers) Thought Disorder– abnormal language and speech. (Schizophrenics use polysyllabic words. Aphasic patients have problems with these complex words.)	Schizophrenia (seen in early 20's)

5
Disorders secondary to Substances

Substance Abuse Disorders
Due to the induction or the use of drugs and substances that cause a disorder. There are several million people in the U.S. with alcoholism and drug abuse. Recreational use does NOT mean immediate addiction. This experimentation may be controlled; however, the problem arises the moment a *dependency* occurs. The dependency signifies a *loss of control* over the use of the substance.
Tolerance indicates that the person need more of a drug to produce the same effect.
Withdrawal effects occur as a reaction when a person abruptly discontinues the use of a substance. Substance abuse is highest among the 18 to 21 year olds, but has the highest risk of abuse is during the period of experimentation (before 16 years old).

Additional risk factors of drug abuse:
Genetic– sons of alcoholics, higher tolerance to alcohol develop into alcoholism (no other abuse with genetic predisposition to known currently); Social– parental difficulties, history of substance abuse, stress, peer pressure, economically disadvantaged, and other "problems".

Overall treatment: Beware of the abuse signs before the abuse happens! This is preventative. The best way to avoid the abuse problem is to teach social skills to prepare for the "experimentation" phase of adolescence and drugs.
Parent groups and drug-prevention campaigns may not be as effective. Detoxification is specific for the drug.
Drug rehabilitation includes stopping drugs, developing social skills, and changing environmental influences (i.e., when trying a cigarette cessation program: throw out **all** the reminders like ash trays, cigarettes, and paraphernalia that have anything that can remind a person of cigarettes.) *Out*patient drug rehabilitation is the BEST choice. Work on the social, family and work issues; keep the motivation to do well, and avoid the reminders. Inpatient drug rehabilitation includes support group therapy, staff counseling, behavioral techniques, and urine drug screens. The recommendation for inpatient rehabilitation is: problems with school-work-

home environments, problems keeping to an outpatient program, associated suicide risk or depression, and legal requirement from a previous court decision. Relapse may occur, and drugs like Disulfiram (Antabuse) are used to avoid the relapse in alcoholism (Methadone is used for heroin addicts, and requires a governmental maintenance program). **Self-help groups** are the **MOST effective treatment** for substance abuse. These include the "12-step" programs, which originated from AA (Alcoholics Anonymous). To cure the person in 12 steps to overcome the problem by using the help of others. Treatment WORKS. The positive response occurs in approximately one half of the treated patients. It takes time, and the more time spent on rehabilitation, the more effective the treatment.

Alcoholism
Alcoholism is a disease. An alcoholic is a person who abuses alcohol and ends up having medical, social, occupational, and/or legal problems. The problems from the consumption of alcohol leads to the disorder. It is not necessarily the amount of drinking. *Heavy* drinkers consume 2-3 drinks/day (but, they may not be an alcoholic since they function normally).
Risk factors: Male, African-American, anti-social personality disorder, mood disorders, waiters, bartenders, and musicians.
Time of onset: Late teens to early 20's.
Alcohol *Abuse*: continued "need" and overindulgence of alcohol that affects the person's life in a social, vocational, educational, or unhealthy way.
Dependence is a physiologic and psychologic need. The *tolerance* develops and requires the person to increase the amount of alcohol (need more to get the same effect) otherwise a *withdrawal syndrome* will occur when it is stopped.
There usually is a positive family history of alcoholism. *Wernicke-Korsakoffs* syndrome is associated with alcohol abuse and decreased nutrition from a lack of thiamine or vitamin B12.

Disulfiram is given to alcoholics in treatment programs to decrease the recurrence of abuse. Disulfiram affects the metabolism of alcohol. It acts by blocking the ***acetaldehyde dehydrogenase***, and increases the acetaldehyde concentration in the blood (toxic effects); this makes the person feel extremely sick when they take alcohol. It is given with the intention that the person will never want to drink again because of how sick it made them (the patient associates illness with drinking).

What happens in **alcohol intoxication**?
Slurred speech, problems with cognition, facial flushing, ataxia, nystagmus, rambling speech, irritability, sadness, and emotional changes (mood swings). Intoxication is based on the *blood alcohol level*. This level varies on the *amount* and *rate* of alcohol consumed, the tolerance level and the body weight. Remember, alcohol is metabolized at the rate of: **1** ounce/*hour*.

How do we treat alcohol intoxication?
The goal is to manage the alcohol abuse and build self-control; decreasing this self-destructive behavior. If blood levels are > 300mg% then, IV Fructose should decrease the level. A normal level will get better in a fairly quick time. Death from alcohol intoxication does not usually occur, UNLESS there is another drug like CNS depressants or sedatives (suicidal person). In diabetics, acidosis or hypoglycemia can result; give the diabetic *Glucose* for treatment. Alcoholics should be placed in rehabilitation programs to effectively treat the alcoholism. Another reason for Detoxification & Rehabilitation programs is for the patient to overcome his drug problem in a setting that does not interfere with the care of other patients in a general psych ward.

What is **alcohol withdrawal**?
It is the symptoms associated with the sudden discontinuance of alcohol consumption:
Course tremors (hands and tongue shake),
Nausea and vomiting,
Weakness,
C-V symptoms: like tachycardia, sweating, HTN and orthostatic hypotension,
Irritability, altered consciousness, and cognitive impairment, and Insomnia.

Usually alcohol withdrawal lasts for a short period and does not risk the life of the individual. BUT, in *Delirium Tremens*, the person has serious hallucinations and other problems ("delirium and trembling") that requires more **physical restraint.** **Diazepam** can initially control delirium (do NOT give neuroleptics). This requires hospitalization. The patient is likely to be vitamin deficient and we administer IM *thiamine*, and B complex **vitamins** to avoid Wernicke-Korsakoff's Syndrome. **Magnesium sulfate** may be given if the patient has significant hypomagnesia (to avoid any seizures).

Alcoholic hallucinosis occurs if the hallucinations stay with the patient even after the delirium has been taken care of.

Wernicke's Syndrome
Delirium with *opthalmoplegia* (abducens nerve-muscle paralysis) and *nystagmus*. There is ataxia, memory loss, altered consciousness, and cognitive impairment (*thiamine* deficiency). Pernicious anemia and malnutrition. Treatment includes: stop the alcohol consumption, give IM thiamine and multivitamins. Delusional ideas include: suspicions, cheating spouse, dishonest relatives, and other delusions. If the delusional ideas persist, then, Neuroleptics may be required.

Drug abuse includes: loss of control over the drug, repeated intoxication, physiologic *tolerance* and social/vocational/economic/or educationally-destructive outcomes.

Drugs of *abuse* include:
* Caffeine and nicotine (coffee and tobacco),
* Alcohol,
Stimulants (cocaine and amphetamines),
Hypnotics and anxiolytics,
Opiates (heroin),
Hallucinogens,
Cannabis (not necessarily *addictive*),
Inhalants.
(*most used and addicting)

Sedative-Hypnotic Overdose
Treatment of an overdose includes: respiratory support and cardiovascular support, **activated charcoal** into the stomach (this will absorb the drugs), sodium bicarbonate infusion (this will alkalinize the urine and increase excretion / decrease reabsorption of phenobarbital). Hemodialysis is done if large amounts of the drug was consumed.

DRUG	**DETOX. TREATMENT**
Meprobamate	IV solution (20%) of Mannitol
Sedative-Hypnotic	IV Naloxone and Glucose; Hemodialysis
Opiates (Heroin) "Snorted" = sniffed into nose "Mainlining" = taken I.V. "Skin popping" = Subcutaneous	Detoxification with: **Methadone** (oral) Maintenance Program Oxygenation, avoid vomitus inhalation, and check C-V function with blood pressure. IV **Naloxone** to counteract the acute effects of opiate intoxication, and to avoid respiratory arrest. Sleep during the withdrawal period can be helped with **Flurazepam**.

DRUG	DETOX. TREATMENT
Cocaine Inhaled = powder, "Free basing" = dissolved in water and smoked. Street cocaine is "cut" with talcum powder or dried milk. "Crack" cocaine = highly potent and pure form; can cause a stroke or cardiac arrest. It gives a quick and intense euphoria.	**Desipramine** (a tricyclic antidepressant) can treat a withdrawal syndrome.

Opiate addiction
Usually seen in African Americans and Hispanic Americans, then by occupation: physicians and nurses! The different types of use are listed above, the street terms are also given for the usage of the drug. The sharing of needles has led to the spread of HIV. Subsequently, heroin addicts are at a substantial risk for **HIV** infection and **AIDS**. The drug causes euphoria, apathy, psychomotor retardation, slurred speech, and poor memory. Usually opiate addicts have a personality disorder, and it is seen with many Vietnam veterans.

Stimulant addiction
Cocaine and amphetamines are stimulants of addiction. Cocaine is a CNS stimulant that is physiologically addictive; "crack" cocaine is highly addictive. It is hard to believe that *millions* of Americans have used cocaine. Cocaine withdrawal is called a "crash". The person is highly anxious and agitated with dysphoria.
Amphetamine and dextroamphetamine are *synthetic* substitutes for ephedrine. Both of the stimulants can cause delusions and hallucinations. Look for: erratic behavior, these individuals are "scanners" (as if looking for some danger).

Hallucinogens
Examples include:
    L S D or *Lysergic acid diethylamide* is an ergot alkaloid derivative. Peyote and mescaline, come from the mescaline cactus.
    THC or Tetrahydrocannabinol (in marijuana) causes euphoria and then drowsiness, it also increases appetite, and causes delusions and visual hallucinations.
    PCP or Phencyclidine causes hostile, bizarre behavior and dissociative anesthesia (insensitivity to pain, with NO loss of consciousness).
    Psilocybin is another hallucinogen.

Hallucinogens are usually used by the upper middle class, and the younger population. The drug affects the perception of visual shapes, colors, and causes the person to "hallucinate". A "bad trip" happens when a person takes a hallucinogen and has a *bad* reaction to it, resulting in permanent brain damage (almost like the movie, *Pulp Fiction*). These abusers end up having psychotic episodes with long-term hallucinations.

Aryl*cyclo*hexylamines
Phencyclidine (PCP) causes intense euphoria with a feeling of incredible power. Phencyclidine inhibits the re-uptake of DA, NE, and 5-IFT. This drug can cause a depression, *psychosis*, and *violent behavior*. It is a white crystalline powder, and looks like cocaine; another name is "angel dust" or "crystal". Like cocaine, it can be snorted, smoked, or injected. This dissociative anesthetic (feel you are not part of your body) causes analgesia and tranquilizes the person with the eyes staying open.

Cannabis or Marijuana
This is the most used illicit (illegal) drug. The active ingredient is tetrahydrocannabinol. "Hashish" is a pure form of cannabis. There is **NO** *physiologic tolerance* to the drug, but there can be *psychological* dependence. The withdrawal syndrome has: anxiety and agitation, tremor, eating disorder and insomnia. Marijuana increases the heart rate and blood pressure, it decreases concentration and impairs the person's ability to learn, decreases the reaction time, and everything appears like it is in slow motion. If the person uses marijuana for a long time, it can affect the lungs and the body's immune system. This increases the risk for infections, lung cancer, and infertility problems. Eventually, *Anti-motivational syndrome* can result, with a loss of interest in doing things.

Inhalants
Predominantly a drug used by poor, usually Latino/Spanish youths. The psychoactive vapors are inhaled from solvents and other chemicals. The intoxication resembles alcohol intoxication but does not last as long. The toxic effects include: delirium, ataxia, tremors, tinnitus (ringing in the ears), and hallucinations.

Substance Abused	Interesting characteristics
Alcohol and Cigarette/chewing Tobacco abuse	Alcohol and cigarette/chewing tobacco abuse is still high, and beginning at a young age. Alcohol is the number one substance of abuse.
Marijuana or cannabis	The number one illicit drug used (but, NO physical addiction).
Cocaine and crack cocaine	Addicts have physical and psychological dependencies with withdrawal problems.
Amphetamines	Euphoric effects. Methamphetamine is also called *Ice*.
Heroin and other Opioids	Isolated behavior develops and problems with anti-social behavior.
PCP or Phencyclidine	"Angel Dust" Hallucinogen causing *violent* behavior.
LSD, Mescaline, Mushrooms (Psilocybin)= Designer Drugs	Illicit labs making drugs that are hallucinogenic; very dangerous.
Inhalants	Glues, paint, nitrous oxide, and gas. Young kids inhale these substances.
Sedative Hypnotics	Benzodiazepines and other hypnotics that cause problems with insomnia.
OTC's (Over-the-Counter's)	Diet pills with dextroamphetamines, antihistamines, and caffeine stimulants.
Steroids	Anabolic steroids used in bodybuilding, can cause excessive anger and have withdrawal effects.

Review:

The substance-related disorders are basically two groups:
    1. The Substance Use Disorders– Substance dependence and abuse.
    2. The Substance-Induced Disorders–   Substance intoxication, withdrawal, delirium, dementia, amnestic, psychotic, mood, anxiety, sexual, and sleep disorders caused by substances.

The Classes of Substances include:
    Alcohol,
    Amphetamines,
    Caffeine,
    Cannabis,
    Cocaine,
    Hallucinogens,
    Inhalants,
    Nicotine,
    Opioids,
    Sedatives,
    and other substances.

6
Schizophrenia & Psychotic Disorders

Schizophrenia
Over half of schizophrenics present *first-rank symptoms* and *hallucinations*, and one-third have *delusional ideas*.

The **negative** features include: *deficits* of thought, speech, and activity. The positive symptoms include: hallucinations and delusions. This leads to the *psychotic* patient who has hallucinations or delusions. The more *negative* features; the *worse* the prognosis ("negative is bad").

Long-term schizophrenia or psychotic patients with few affective symptoms and many negative features do worse. The long-term outcome for *schizoaffective disorder* is better. Males (begin at 21 years old) show signs earlier than females (begin at 27). Male to Female ratio is *equal*. Males chronic. *Downward drift* results. Diagnosis of schizophrenia includes: presentation of psychotic features (delusions or hallucinations), few affective disorders, and no history or examination of coarse brain disease, and young adulthood onset of the illness. Do NOT look for lab results, there are NO *pathognomonic* lab results of schizophrenia (just some abnormal lab tests).

Schizophrenia comes from damage or influences like: infection, neural developmental problems, head trauma, and the use of illicit drugs. The genetic predisposition possibly needs this irritation to express the schizophrenia. Family history is important, schizophrenia is familial, and is seen more in first-degree relatives (like parents, brothers, or children). **Mono**zygotic twins have a higher risk of developing schizophrenia than dizygotic twins (of relatives with schizophrenia).

Treatment includes: periodic hospitalization, eventual institutionalization or maintaining a structured environment, hospitalization for medically unresponsive psychotic symptoms. Change the individuals behavior by creating a direct, reality-oriented environment (comments are real). Show a calm, supportive environment to decrease anxiety and increase compliance. Drug of choice includes: Neuroleptics to decrease the psychotic symptoms. Long term: Over half will regain social abilities, but NOT a *complete* remission.

Schizophrenia (continued)

Haloperidol is the most commonly used neuroleptic for psychosis (20-40mg/ day).
Chlorpromazine.
Adding **Lithium** to the neuroleptic treatment may help.
Fluphenazine is also used. IM or intramuscular form of Haloperidol or Fluphenazine is given to maintain the dose in the non-compliant patients (this will allow over 2 weeks to go by between treatments).
ECT is considered on patients resistant to antipsychotics.
Clozapine has also been used. (Remember pharmacology: the association of *agranulocytosis* with clozapine; therefore, use this drug last.)
Maintain on medication for over a half a year. **Risk** of treatment include: **Tardive dyskinesia**. Therefore, discontinue the neuroleptics after a year. Anti-Parkinsonian drugs may be used if the extrapyramidal symptoms are severe.

Most schizophrenics do no harm. They do NOT cause problems to others. The problem is with the *lack of* interest and poor care of themselves. They are improperly dressed, loiter in hallways, cause burns because of smoking; and just doing nothing! This is why hospital staff has to be trained to take care of patients and reward positive behaviors.

Better prognosis in schizophrenia is associated with:
    A calm family (less emotional expression or less emotional excitement),
    Acute onset,
    A later onset,
    Females.

Psychosis

Impaired ability to recognize reality. This leads to irregular behavior and creativity. Psychotic patient must have one or more of the following: Hallucinations, delusions, irregular speech pattern, and disorganized behavior.

Hallucination	Sensing (visual, auditory, tactile, taste, or smell) something that has NO real external stimulus.
Delusion	A false belief; from an actual external stimulus, but of incorrect understanding and no proof.

Overview of Psychotic Disorders:

Schizophrenia	Lasts for 6 months or more. With psychotic symptoms for at least 1 month. Treatment = antipsychotics and social therapy.
Schizophreniform Disorder	Like schizophrenia, but, it lasts for *less than* 6 months. Can be thought of as "acute schizophrenia" since it lasts for 1 to 6 months. Treatment = antipsychotics and social therapy.
Schizoaffective Disorder	Having both Psychotic features *and* Mood symptoms. Treatment = Mood stabilizing meds (Lithium, antidepressants, and ECT) and antipsychotics.
Delusional Disorder	Having persistent delusions, but NO psychotic features. This is Paranoia. These people are not really bizarre. Treatment = Antipsychotics for the delusions, and anxiolytics.
Brief Psychotic Disorder	Sudden psychosis of < 1 month. Usually after a serious stressful event, and then the person will go back to normalcy. This is seen with postpartum women.
Shared Psychotic Disorder	When the psychotic behaviors are also believed by a person with a close relationship. (shares the other person's delusion) Treatment = antipsychotics.
Substance-Induced Psychosis	Psychosis from a drug, but with NO delirium nor dementia. Treatment = remove the causative agent, and treat the drug withdrawal.

Schizophrenia Subtypes

Catatonia type	Active Schizophrenic phase with catatonia. (Immobility, stupor, excessive motor activity, peculiar postures, or echolalia may be present)
Disorganized type	NO catatonia, but the person is disorganized (disorganized speech, behavior, and flat affect).
Paranoid type	Hallucinating or having delusions. (NOT catatonic nor disorganized)
Undifferentiated type	Active Schizophrenic phase, but not one of the above three types.
Residual type	NO active phase. No prominent delusions or hallucinations, but there are negative symptoms or odd beliefs.

Schizo*affective* Disorder
Psychotic behavior with no coarse brain disease. (These persons are between schizophrenia and a mood disorder.) There is a period of major depression or mania (*affective* disorder) with the symptoms of *schizophrenia*.

Schizophreniform Disorder
Schizophrenia criteria lasting between 1 to 6 months, but not longer.

Delusional Disorder
Includes *paranoia* (or "insanity"), *with* delusional ideas. If there are no hallucinations but there are delusions, we call it *simple* delusional disorder. A person has one delusional idea but no other problems in decreased personality traits.
Paraphrenia is a mild form of delusions that shows up in adulthood or retirement age (unlike schizophrenia that happens in young adulthood). Paranoid person is hypersensitive, always suspicious, and jealous. They tend to find blame in people. Usually seen in males, around 40-50 years old and married. They do NOT develop into schizophrenia.
Induced psychotic disorder is a delusion that is formed because of another person who has the delusional idea (by hanging out with a person, believe their delusion).

Delusions
A false or awkward idea with no proof. Delusional ideas may come from an altered mood like euphoria or sadness that changes the thinking and creates false generalizations. In euphoria, the person feels "on top of the world" and maybe the "leader". Other times, the patient feels things are real, and supports the delusion by making reference to "voices warning against danger...*real* voices" when actually they are hallucinations. Delusions occur in affective disorder, coarse brain disease, and schizophrenia; they are not pathognomonic of one disorder.

Primary **delusional idea**
When a delusion appears without any other psychopathology. *Autochthonous* delusional idea (a type of primary delusional idea) forms abruptly. The delusional conclusions are false, and have no logic (the delusional idea comes from illogical thinking), but they are based on real perceptions (i.e., a person believes that a store manager is going to kill him because the light bulb is out). It is *primary* whenever there is no other psychopathology present.

Secondary **delusional idea**
When a delusion comes from another psychopathology; because it came second, and may have been derived from the first psychopathology.

Mood-congruent idea (a type of secondary delusional idea) appears *from* an altered *mood*.

Mood-incongruent ideas (secondary and primary delusional ideas) came from psychopathology **not** related to mood changes.

Delusional mood
The delusional feeling or experience. "Something *terrible* is happening; I don't know what it is..."

Perceptions
Hallucinations do not have any outside stimuli. Hallucinations happen with all senses: visual (i.e., seeing things), auditory (hearing voices), olfactory (smelling odors), gustatory (tasting), tactile (feeling spiders), and visceral ("something inside of me pushing out"). Non-pathologic conditions: having hallucinations when a person is exhausted or is falling asleep. *Illusions* are misinterpretations of actual outside stimuli.

Psychosensory Symptoms

Seen in *partial epilepsy*, schizophrenia, and mood disorders. Temporo-limbic dysfunction. Treatment may include: Valproic acid or Carbamazepine.

Psychosensory Symptom	Definition / Example
Autonomic Paroxysms	"I feel very cold." or "My heart is beating very fast." (Bodily changes without being frightened or exercising.)
Depersonalization	"I was floating above and I could see myself. " (detachment from self)
Derealization	"Nothing around me seems to be here, am I in a dream?" (Person feels to be in an environment that is not real, like walking in a dream. Things seem to be occurring without them.)
Deja vu	"It feels like I've been here before." (Familiarity; feeling of being, doing, or saying something before; even though it is really the first time)
Dysacousia	"I can't hear any train." (when it is very apparent) or "I can hear the conversation from here." (when there is no way to) Impaired hearing but no actual loss of hearing perception.
Emotional incontinence.	Expresses emotions at the smallest events. (Patient cries just because he sees a sad face.)
Jamais vu	"It feels like I've *never* been here before." (Not recognizing a location, person or experience that you have commonly been to. *Un*familiarity. Opposite of deja vu.)
Visceral hallucinations	"Something inside of me", "A knife pushing out of my stomach."

First-Rank Symptoms of Schneider
In schizophrenia and affective disorder patients (manics), the 11 first-rank symptoms (seen in approx. 75% of schizophrenics) include: thought broadcasting, experiences of influence, experiences of alienation, complete auditory hallucinations (most common symptom), and delusional perceptions. To be a first-rank symptom, the control must be felt physically, be irresistible, and be delusional (bizarre or unbelievable).

First-Rank Symptoms	Characteristics
Thought broadcasting	Patient experiences his thoughts leaving his head. "Others can hear what I am thinking." Controlled by something outside.
Experiences of Influence	"Stop looking at me like that, I know you are trying to X-ray me with your eyes."
Experiences of Alienation	No longer feeling self. Now, part of someone else. Parts of their body, like the right leg wasn't their leg.
Complete Auditory Hallucinations	Hearing voices. Coming from a few people, and possibly re-stating the patient's thoughts. This is called "thought echo". Most common symptom.
Delusional Perceptions	"I feel warmth under my skin."

Brief Reactive Psychosis
A stressful event brings on an instant psychosis. The person is emotionally labile and moody. Once the problem is removed, the person is "cured".

Postpartum Psychosis
Women are at highest risk for psychiatric illness during the first weeks *after* childbirth (psychosis is highest after the delivery of that ugly baby!). Actually, it is due to the change in hormones and body function; the serum *progesterone* levels drop. Postpartum psychosis usually happens from the first pregnancy. Mood disorder and depression are the most frequent problems. Mania may arise, and the person acts disoriented and delusional.

Drug-induced Psychosis
Psychosis that is caused by drugs, like: Lysergic acid diethylamide (LSD), mescaline, Psilocybin, dimethyltryptamine (DMT), phencyclidine (PCP), cannabis, amphetamines, and cocaine. Treatment includes: lithium or neuroleptics, acidifying the urine, and ECT if medications do not work. In amphetamine psychosis: use Haloperidol. In PCP psychosis: acidify the urine (use *ammonium chloride*) and add Furosemide (Lasix) to increase the excretion of the drug.

Neuroleptic Malignant Syndrome (NMS)
NMS extrapyramidal side effects, hyperthermia and then catatonia. Treatment includes: neuroleptics, a dopamine agonist (like Bromocriptine), and a muscle relaxant (like Dantrolene or Lorazepam).

7
Mood Disorders

Mood Disorders
Problems with mood. Previous name was *Organic mental disorders*. Now, an organic mental disorder is called a *Mood Disorder due to a General medical condition*. Depression (unhappy/sad mood), and mania (elevated mood) or bipolar disorder (manic-depressive) are examples of mood disorders. Disorders are due to a general medical condition include: Delirium, dementia, Amnestic disorder, psychotic disorder, catatonic disorder, mood disorder, anxiety disorder, sexual dysfunction, sleep disorder, and personality change– all due to a general *medical* condition. Substance induced mental disorders also occur.

Melancholia
An overwhelming feeling of sadness or despair that preoccupies the persons mind. *Dysphoria* is the combination of melancholia *and* irritability. Melancholics are worried or overwhelmed and confused. They have mood swings, and insomnia (often wake up early). Often with anorexia and suicidal thoughts, with feelings of hopelessness and guilt. Look for the sad facial appearances like the *omega sign* (look for "Ω" between the eyebrows) and Veraguth's folds (see illustration below).

The Omega Sign   *Veraguth's folds*

Melancholic individuals have repetitive movements and show their agitation by their hand movements and rubbing; sometimes with self-destructive behavior. They possibly have problems with their neuroendocrine system and the hypothalamus. These lead to changes in *circadian rhythms* and the body's functions, like the: cycles of the body temperature, sleep-wake cycle, menstruation, growth hormones and cortisol. Changes with a person's appetite (decreased), heart rate and perspiration.

Melancholia (continued)
Consider hospitalizing a melancholic patient if there are suicidal thoughts, anorexia, stupor, or psychosis. Tell the patient that this problem is biologic, and is not a something that a person can voluntarily control. With treatment, they will most likely have a good response and be back to their old self. Increase the family support and be aware of suicidal tendency. Weigh the patient every day (to see if they are improving their diet).

ECT, tricyclic antidepressants, and lithium are the treatments. ECT is the treatment of choice for inpatient settings. Otherwise, a tricyclic antidepressant, or combine a TCA with a MAOI. If the melancholic person is *bipolar*, treat with *lithium* or combine with a MAOI.

Psychotic Depression
Periods of depression *with* delusions or hallucinations.
> Mood congruent
> *Depressive* content. The delusions are compatible with mood disorders. Treatment: Tricyclic antidepressants.
>
> Mood **in**congruent
> *Persecutory* content or a first-rank symptom. More compatible with schizophrenia. Treatment: MAOI's.
>
> Treatment: ECT has the fewest side effects and a good response to treatment. With drug therapy use: lithium or lithium with carbamazepine or a monoamine oxidase inhibitor (MAOI). Use antidepressants with neuroleptics. (With the risks of tardive dyskinesia, neuroleptics may actually want to be avoided.)

***Non*melancholic Depression**
Don't hospitalize atypical depression. Treatment includes: a tricyclic antidepressant or MAOI *with psychotherapy*.

Dysthymia
Depressed mood with poor appetite or binge eating, insomnia or hypersomnia, poor concentration and fatigue, and feelings of hopelessness. This disorder is *like* major depression, but there has NOT been a depressive or manic episode. It is a *chronic* problem, and there are NO hallucinations or other problems like delusions.

***Reactive* Depression**
Depression that occurs after an known environmental stresser or a precipitating event.

Neurotic **depression**
Similar to reactive depression and slightly like dysthymia.

Depressive pseudodementia
Seen in older individuals with melancholia and cognitive problems, and concentration problems. Look for *dementia* with: weight loss, insomnia, other cognitive problems, *and melancholia*. (This is NOT Alzheimer's, because of these extra signs.)

Lab Testing in depression
The Sedation Threshold Test
Barbiturates will sedate, and the endogenous depressives are sensitive to I.V. barbiturates. Reactive depressives are NOT sensitive to the sedatives.

Dexamethasone Suppression Test
A *positive* test means the depressed person most likely has *endogenous* depression. (Practically NO *reactive* depressives have a positive test.)

Acute mania
This is a medical emergency. The person is excited, hyperactive, and is assaultive. Treatment: give a *neuroleptic*, and isolate the person if he gets out of control. Haloperidol (20-30 mg), given IM in the *gluteal* muscle; twice a day for two days. This is given until the person is stabilized, then Lithium is given. If there is no response to the neuroleptic treatment, then ECT treatments are given for 3 days. Manics need at least 8 ECT treatments (and more ECT's than depressives) to avoid a recurrence.

Hypomania
When a patient is not *extremely* excited or assaultive and can take oral medication (he is very close to being manic). Lithium is the treatment. Take the Lithium levels two times a week until the therapeutic level is maintained. Problems getting to the therapeutic level include: the patient is not compliant and is not taking the medication; polyuria can also excrete the drug; or the dose needs to be increased. Remember, Lithium has an anti-diuretic hormone (ADH) effect and causes a great volume of excretion of urine and the drug.

Lithium
If the patient is hypomanic or manic, *Lithium* is the first drug of choice. If the person becomes out of control– a *Neuroleptic* is the drug of choice (give IM Haloperidol and then oral Haloperidol). (Or carbamazepine or valproic acid). Always check the renal, liver, and thyroid functions; and take a drug level.

Mood disorders are familial. Higher rates of mood disorder is seen in biologic relatives, and an *increased* **dopa**minergic function in *mania*, and *decreased* **seroton**ergic function in *depression*. This represents the biochemical problem. Depression has a deficiency of serotonin, and mania has an excess of dopamine (Catecholamine hypothesis).

Bipolar Affective Disorder

Depression *with* episodes of mania or hypomania. Must have depression *and* mania to be considered *bipolar*. The manic person feels: euphoria, hyperactive, has pressured speech, grandiose feelings and flight of ideas. Mood is elevated or the person can be irritated and emotionally labile. Problems with attention and concentration, they are easily distracted, they are **un**inhibited (they are the "King of the hill" and have no shame). Problems with the frontal lobe possible, but with adequate treatment, the person can function normally.

Other Conditions:

Suicide

Greater number of suicide attempts than actual death from suicide. Highest risk after attempting suicide.
Males die from suicide 4x more than women. (Highest > 45 years old)
Women *attempt* suicide 4x more than men. (due to less violent attempts, like drugs and wrist slashing, while men use guns, etc.) (Highest > 55 years old)
#3 cause of death in young adults (accidents, homicide, then suicide).
Most important risk factor for suicide: an *intent to commit* suicide.
Increased risk factors: Depression, physicians (psychiatrists are the highest!), police officers, dentists, lawyers, musicians, divorced male > female, unmarried (marriage is good...), > 45 years old, white > black, drug abuse history, history of psychiatric illness, Jewish or Protestants > Catholic individuals. Major depression is associated with death by *suicide*. Alcoholism is also associated with suicide. Suicide is greater for Native Americans. (But, NO difference in suicide and *income*). Protestants commit suicide more than Catholics (it's a bad sin, so Catholics don't commit as much suicide). Although, at a time of economic stress, suicide risk rises. Keep your eyes open for indications of possible suicide: previous suicide attempt, person may have no support at home or work, depression, family history, physical illness, etc.
Most common method of suicide: Firearms (65% of total suicides), poisoning, and hanging/strangulation.
ECT is a useful treatment for major depressive episodes. Medication management: Tricyclic antidepressants are preferred (NOT barbiturates). A large portion (as much as half) of the suicides are by overdose with drugs prescribed by a physician.

Lethal catatonia
The sudden intense excitement of mania and delirium, with catatonic features, and high fever in a patient who was in good health. ECT is lifesaving (and may go into remission).

Cyclothymia
Mood disorder that has mood swings from excitement to depression (but do NOT meet the criteria for depression or other disorder). A cyclothymic person usually has an endomorphic body type, the person is extroverted and outgoing, BUT, the person is impulsive and has a labile mood.

Late-Luteal Phase Syndrome = Premenstrual Syndrome (PMS)
PMS is now called: Late-luteal phase syndrome. It usually begins in the mid-30's. The problems in this syndrome are: water retention, discomfort, impulsiveness, depression, and problems with social life. There is a higher chance for major depression than in women without PMS.

Bereavement
Reaction to the recent loss of a loved one; has the symptoms of major depression like poor appetite and insomnia. "Normal" bereavement or grief can last a couple of months (it varies with different cultures), and support is the best treatment. BUT, it is considered **ab**normal if it lasts over **2** months. At this point, the diagnosis of *major depressive* episode can be made.

Secondary Depression
Some common causes of secondary depression are: aging, systemic diseases like lupus erythematosus (SLE), stroke, basal ganglia disease, head trauma, aging, and multiple sclerosis.

Laboratory Findings
Lab results in mood disorders are similar to schizophrenia. In schizophrenics and depressives, we see *ventricular enlargement*. CT's of manics show: enlarged *lateral* ventricles, and cerebellar atrophy. MRI show: decreased frontal lobe size in bipolar patients and the older depressed patients. Small temporal lobe size in bipolar patients, and decreased caudate size in depressed patients. Neuroendocrine findings in patients with mood disorders also have clinical implications. [Dexamethasone Suppression Test (DST): take the plasma cortisol levels in the morning, in the afternoon, and late evening; and *increased* level is **ab**normal. Melancholic persons are **non**suppressors. Otherwise, consider Cushing's disease or another systemic illness. Thyrotropin Releasing Hormone (TRH): after an overnight fast, a *low* TSH (*stimulating* hormone) level is **ab**normal; consider a mood disorder or melancholia. DST and TRH measure the hypothalamic-pituitary function.]

Some mood disorders show recurrent episodes that appear to be cyclical in nature, or of a particular pattern of occurrence. There may be a full remission in between episodes or partial remission.

This can include:

Seasonal Pattern
An onset of episodes of depression during a certain time of the year. Usually depression occurs in the later part of the year; in the Fall or in the Winter. This is followed by remission periods in other times of the year; Spring is uplifting!

Rapid-Cycling Pattern
Episodes that occur and go into partial or full remission, and switch. This happens at least 4 times a year.

8
Anxiety Disorders

Cognitive Anxiety and Somatic Anxiety
Cognitive anxiety is when the person over-worries about an event and forms insecure feelings and stress (can be considered "worry warts"). These patients tend to have poor recovery after an illness. They are *low* novelty seekers and have *low* reward dependency, and they have high harm avoidance. Treatment: anxiolytics or other anti-anxiety therapies can be helpful.

Somatic anxiety occurs when the person feels disturbed, easily distracted, and develops aches and pains or other nervous symptoms. They are *High* novelty seekers and have *High* reward dependency, and they have *low* harm avoidance (all opposite from cognitive anxiety). Treatment: No real treatment received from anti-anxiety drugs; other forms of behavioral modification may help.

Anxiety disorders: simple and social *phobias* do not *run* in families; but, the other anxiety disorders are familial.

Neurosis was the term used for anxiety disorder.

Panic attack
A period of anxiety that overwhelm the individual. *Respiratory **alkalosis*** may occur as a result of the patient *hyper*ventilating. Treatment includes: Anxiolytics like *Diazepam* or *Chlordiazepoxide*.

Panic disorder
Having a sudden panic or anxiety attack, or an overwhelming sense of doom; problems breathing, and fear of death. They respond with physiologic changes as if there was a real threat; the pupils dilate the sympathetic flight-or-fight response happens for about 30 minutes. The panic attack can continue to a point where the patient becomes overwhelmed, and unable to function. Diagnosis is based on at least 4 panic attacks in a 4 month period of time, and a fear of having another attack (lasts for a month). For diagnosis, administering IV **sodium lactate** will *induce* a panic attack in anxiety patients. Sodium lactate or **bicarbonate** can induce panic attacks in anxiety disorders.

Phobias
When the person has an **ir**rational fear of some situation. The actual danger is not there, but the patient is fearful as if there was danger (i.e., a fear of heights and falling, but there is a steel railing that will not allow even a child to fall). The most common phobias include fears of: animals/insects, situations (heights), and blood / physical damage. Simple *phobic* disorder presents differently than simple *panic* disorder. Since the *phobia* begins in *childhood* (i.e., phobia of school). [While, simple *panic* disorder and agoraphobia begin in the **20**'s; *Never* before puberty or after 35]. Agoraphobic patients become more isolated and undergo serious social and work problems. Eventually becoming "housebound". *Irritable bowel syndrome* and *mitral valve prolapse* are associated with these anxiety disorders. The most common problem associated with this anxiety is: *depression*. Treatment includes: Tricyclic antidepressants, MAOI's, and if the patient has bipolar affective disorder: lithium, anticonvulsants, or ECT.

Agoraphobia
Fear of leaving home and going to the outside; these people are often intelligent, but are fearful of leaving their home, so they remain inside for up to years without going out. The panic disorder occurs with agoraphobia because of the panic attack when they try to go out. These panic attacks occur while the person is separated from home. Usually women will hyperventilate, and have a panic attack when going away from their home.

Obsessional Syndromes
Repetitive, intrusive thoughts and actions. The problems include:
>Obsessive compulsive disorder (OCD)
>Gilles de la Tourette's syndrome (GTS or Tourette's Disorder)
>Trichotillomania (pulling hair)
>Hypochondriasis if there is only one or a few recurrent health issues
>Anorexia nervosa
>Post-traumatic stress disorder (PTSD)
>Sexual disorders like exhibitionism

Obsessive-Compulsive Disorder
Obsessions: "obsessive" or recurrent thoughts/impulses that the patient sees as meaningless, but he can't resist and must do it. *Compulsions*: repetitive, "ritualistic" acts, usually compelled by obsessive thoughts. Just because the person does the ritual, does not mean he is satisfied. Obsessive-Compulsive Disorder types:
>Handwashers, Checkers, Orderers, Repeaters, and
>Pure obsessionals (only have thoughts and impulses but No rituals).

Obsessive-Compulsive Disorder (continued)
They form anxiety with *fear of contamination* that "can harm". Usually first seen over 16 years old and early 20s (but, *never* > 35). OCD patients have abnormal personalities, they are: passive-aggressive, avoidant or dependent. There is a *familial* basis and a genetic origin. It can occur as a result of problems with: frontal lobe or limbic system; as a result of *carbon monoxide poisoning*. Biochemically, serotonin is the neurotransmitter involved in such repetitive and impulsive behaviors; an increase in 5-HT may be seen in OCD. The treatment is geared to decrease the obsessive and compulsive drives of the individual. OCD symptoms are reduced by Mocking the reuptake of serotonin (SSRI's = Serotonin-selective reuptake inhibitors). The SSRI drug of choice is: *Clomipramine* (Anafranil). Fluoxetine (Prozac) is also used, and Buspirone (minimal sedation). Neuroleptics (like Haloperidol) are used on patients who are resistant to SSRI's and who have *tics*.

Gilles de la Tourette's (GTS)
Tourette's Syndrome is a disorder of vocal and motor tics, coprolalia (sudden foul language; i.e., "sh_t" repeated quickly), and echolalia. Usually seen in Whites (Not in Blacks), and Males. Starts as a child up until about 16 years old. In this disorder we find characteristics like: *tics, repetitive movements, echolalia* and *echoprasia*. **Tics** occur with: the *eyes, vocalizations* (pathologic coughing, barking, throat clearing; making irregular sounds), and coprolalia (uncontrolled swearing). **Repetitive movements** include: hitting, touching, and stamping feet. It is also associated with self-injurious behavior and sleep disorders. Familial, and usually seen in males. GTS has compulsions, and family history of tics. Both have an early age of onset, lifetime symptoms come and go, these are unwanted behaviors, and therefore is similar to Obsessive-Compulsive Disorder. The treatment includes: *Haloperidol* or *Clomipramine (Anafranil)*, and behavioral therapy.

Generalized anxiety disorder (GAD)
Anxiety with**out** panic or phobic disorders.

Post-Traumatic Stress Disorder (PTSD)
A stressful event in the person's life that causes stress in related circumstances or at random. The common stressful events include: automobile accidents, rape victims, war, or other major catastrophe. The common term, "shell shock" from the first World War is an example. These patients usually have other existing problems like: alcohol and drug abuse, antisocial personality, obsessive-compulsive disorder, anxiety, or depression.

Treatment for Anxiety Disorders:
Tricyclic antidepressants, MAOIs, and benzodiazepines; then, beta-blockers and anticonvulsants. These treatments are effective because of the changes in the neurotransmitters in anxiety disorders: *increased* norepinephrine, *decreased* GABA (not enough inhibition of thoughts), or serotonergic. The medications work on these transmitters and are helpful.

> **Tricyclic Antidepressants** are successful for the treatment of: panic disorder, generalized anxiety disorder, and agoraphobia. Imipramine for panic disorder. **SSRI**'s like **Fluoxetine (Prozac)** for anxiety disorders. Gradually increase the dosage to reach the therapeutic level with these drugs.
> **Monoamine Oxidase Inhibitors (MAOI's)**
> > **Phenelzine** MAOI for anxiety disorders.
>
> First try the tricyclic antidepressants. There are side effects with MAOI's and the patient needs to avoid foods with *tyramine* (they have to be on a restricted diet). A hypertensive reaction may occur. You can add a MAOI to antidepressants, but don't add antidepressants to MAOI because the patient can become delirius and go into an *adrenergic crisis*. Sublingual *Nifedipine* will correct a hypertensive reaction. *Phentolamine* or *Prazosin* will treat a tyramine-induced hypertension.
> **Benzodiazepines**
> These are important drugs, and considered the drug of choice for acute *panic attacks*. Treatment for anxiety disorders. But, they have addictive properties so give tricyclic antidepressants and MAOI's. The benzodiazepines have an anti-anxiety effect because of the GABA action.
> > **Alprazolam** is a *high*-potency drug that is used for panic disorder. It is short-acting drug that needs to be given T.I.D. (3 times per day).
> > Clonazepam and Lorazepam. Clonazepam is *intermediate*-acting and is given B.I.D. (2 times per day)

Cognitive Behavior Therapy
Behavior therapy given by psychologists. This is best if given in conjunction with drugs. This is the best form of therapy for *simple phobias*. Anxiety disorders can get better when combined with drug therapy. The patient is treated by increasing exposures to anxiety-provoking thoughts and situations that may provoke an anxiety attack. The person runs through *imagery* (thinking about a difficult situation) and exposure to the situation.

Neurosurgery is also possible for unresponsive cases; there are minimal side effects, but risks associated with surgery. The theory is that the hippocampus, amygdala, and parahippocampus increase the uptake after a sodium lactate infusion. The temporal lobe seems to be involved with panic disorder.

9
Somatoform & Factitious Disorders

Somatoform Disorders
These include: somatization (hysteria and Briquet's syndrome), hypochondriasis, somatoform pain disorder, and body dysmorphic disorder.

Somatization disorder
Appears as a bunch of symptoms affecting the person, but having NO medical basis (the results of lab and clinical findings show no pathology).
Briquet's syndrome– histrionic personality that affects the body, and the person complains of every problem known to man. It's all in the mind, and there are no lab or clinical findings to support the complaints of the patient. Treatment: tell the patient that she has Briquet's Syndrome and that it will improve; a placebo affect is possible.

This begins in early teens, but never after age 30. It is usually seen with *women*. The patient has **10** or more symptoms that cannot be documented by medical knowledge. Somatization symptoms include: feeling sick, pseudoneurologic problems, C-V, G-I and G-U problems, impotence, and irregular pain.

To diagnose somatization disorder, the examiner can ask if there are any of the following: vomiting, problems with swallowing / shortness of breath / burning sensations, dysmennorhea or other pain. Two or more symptoms in men and three or more symptoms in women are suggestive of the disorder. Treatment: NONE, let the patient know that NO medicine is *good* medicine in this case.

Conversion disorder
A disorder that recognizes neurologic disorders, but it is really *pseudo*neurologic (have the signs and symptoms or neurologic disorders, but no tests can validate them– no EEG, CT, or MRI findings of irregularities or lesions). The tests performed include: EEG, CT, or MRI of the CNS, LP (lumbar puncture), EMG (electromyography), and sensory evoked potentials. [Multiple sclerosis can be caught with these tests.]

Signs and symptoms can include: paralysis, seizures, aphasia, problems with coordination blindness, and anesthesia. Pseudocyesis = mistaken pregnancy

Conversion disorder (continued)
(the *conversion* of a desire or fear of pregnancy into actual physical symptoms like not having the menstrual period, scaring the husband that she is pregnant, and even lactating!). But, pregnancy or prolactinomas can cause the symptoms, and a regular evaluation is expected. This disorder is more common in *women*, and low socioeconomic levels.

The belief is that there is a *conflict* between a desire and a fear of that want and this converts into *physical* symptoms; thus the name, *soma*tization.

Many conversion signs are on the body's *left* side, and may have *right* hemisphere problems. Conversion disorder should be taken seriously because the person could have a serious medical or psychiatric problem.

Somatoform pain disorder
Chronic pain (somatoform pain) that causes impairment in social or occupational functions. *Sympathetic* nervous system problems can be misdiagnosed as somatoform pain; thermography must be done.

Hypochondriasis
Overreacting to or making normal signs symptoms abnormal. The person (usually a women) becomes preoccupied with having a life-threatening disease. It is always *secondary to* another problem like depression or obsessive-compulsive disorder.

Body dysmorphic disorder
The preoccupation with a body part or an organ. The patient may have a problem with the lower colon or the ear lobes, etc.

Factitious Disorder

When a person makes up symptoms and deliberately shows physical signs. *Factitious illness* is intentionally creating physical signs (fraud is NOT a part of factitious illness).

Malingering

When a person makes up symptoms and deliberately shows physical signs. *Malingering* is producing fake symptoms with **fraud** in mind. They are interested in some form of financial gain or compensation, or they are avoiding obligations (like military duty). It is usually associated with: antisocial personality, drug and alcohol addiction. The most common symptoms given are: hallucinations and suicide, anxiety, and post-traumatic stress disorder. Some systemic illness by falsely heating a thermometer (get out of school), they may drink something hot to increase the temperature, self-destructive behavior, just faking anything they can come up with. Confront the patient firmly or discharge the patient.

10
Dissociative Disorders

Dissociative States
Coarse brain disorder caused by: amnesia, intoxication, epilepsy, and CNS infection.

Dissociative Amnesia
Was called psychogenic amnesia in the past. These patients are unable to recall personal information. Caused by trauma or stress, and is NOT ordinary forgetfulness.

Dissociative Fugue
Was called psychogenic fugue in the past. It is the sudden travel away from home or work and not recalling the person's past. The person suddenly leaves home for hours or several days, is confused, and may assume a new identity.

Depersonalization Disorder
Feelings of being "outside of my body" or feel "like I am in a dream." These persons can reality test, but they have recurrent episodes that interfere with work or school.

Dissociative Identity Disorder
Was called Multiple personality disorder in the past. Having 2 or more personalities and forgetting personal identity. This disorder is NOT secondary to drugs or medical conditions.

> "We must be courageous, but also reasonable. The world admires us for walking a tightrope without falling off. It asks us to keep our balance."
> —Lech Walesa

You are half way through with your Psychiatry book, it's time for a short break. Take a moment and stretch out, Congratulations thus far!

11
Sexual & Gender Identity Disorders

Sexually Deviant Behavior
Freud related *deviant* behavior to *psycho*sexual development. The irregular behavior may be a limbic system dysfunction. *Homo*sexuality is considered an alternate form of sexual behavior, and is NOT considered pathologic. Sexual deviations include:
Sexual dysfunctions (problems with arousal and performance)
Paraphilias (inappropriate or dangerous sexual behaviors)
Gender identity disorders (childhood and or adolescent conditions)

Sexual dysfunction
This includes disorders of: Arousal, Desire, Sexual orgasm, and Pain.
*Hypo*sexuality is *decreased* sexual arousal and activity. Many of the drugs used in medicine and especially psychiatry affect the sexual function of the individual. This is associated with the *anticholinergic* properties which affects the sexual ability. *Hyper*sexuality is *increased* sexual arousal and activity. It is associated with *mania*. The sexual behavior can extend into verbal and manipulative public display like masturbation or fondling.
Sexual aversion disorder is the recurrent aversion or dislike of sex.
Kleine-Levin Syndrome is the hypothalamic problem of hypersexuality with hyperphagia (too much sex and food needs).

Kluver-Bucy Syndrome
Lack of sexual inhibition with visual agnosia. Occurs with Pick's disease and Alzheimer's disease as a result of: *bilateral hippocampal or temporal degeneration.* The hypersexuality shows as increased oral needs, agnosia, and cognitive problems. Personality traits (NOT disorders) of sexual extremes include: *satyriasis* and *nymphomania*.

Other problems of sexual function:
Premature ejaculation, pain during sexual intercourse (dyspareunia), and painful vaginal contractions (vaginismus) preclude or interrupt penetration. This is usually the result of personality disorders, anxiety disorders, or stressful situations. *Impotence* or the inability to have an erection, can also occur because of systemic disease; like, diabetes, and substance abuse.

Treatment: ruling out a systemic or neurologic problem, the deviant sexual behavior is treated with drug and behavioral therapy. Behavioral therapy: Relaxation techniques and desensitization. Treatment is geared to involving both partners. This decreases the anxiety and increases the response.
For vaginismus: Vaginal dilators or using fingers to dilate the vagina.
For premature ejaculation: The squeeze technique (the partner usually squeezes the head of the penis and prevents ejaculation)

Paraphilias are treated with behavioral techniques and social skills training. Medications like: *anti-androgenic libido suppressants* (Medroxyprogesterone) or Cyproterone (Androcur) are used to inhibit the androgens at the receptors. The idea is that by reducing the sexual hormones and the testosterone levels, this will decrease the sexual drive.

Paraphilias
Frequent strong sexual urge/fantasy focused on inanimate *objects, children* and any person refusing the assault (Although, *rape* is **not** a paraphilia). This is why paraphilias are usually considered *hetero*sexual acts. Coarse brain disease can cause the paraphilia.
Paraphilias include: Exhibitionism, Masochism, Sadism, Transvestism, Fetishism, and Pedophilia.

Gender identity disorders
Transsexualism
The overwhelming need to change the sexual characteristics and anatomy of the person because of a belief that the person is really of the opposite sex. (These individual feels to be in the body of the wrong sex gender.) They have sex-change operations because they are always feeling uncomfortable with their gender (he appears as a man, but he wants to be a women), and he is preoccupied with gaining the opposite sexual characteristics. Transsexuals can be asexual, homosexual, or heterosexual. If the patient has surgery, they are almost always happy with the appearance and change (since they have always felt like being the opposite sex, they do very well and can even go on to become famous models like James Bond's girl; so, it may be recommended to help the person adjust). The downside of surgery is usually that it was**n't** *enough* of the secondary sexual characteristics to feel like the opposite sex.
[**Transvestism** is cross-dressing; to look like the other sex, and they are usually *hetero*sexual)

Neurological or systemic disorders (like epilepsy), an anxiety disorder or OCD (they are obsessed with becoming the opposite sex), and anti-social personality can cause the sexual disorientation.

12
Eating Disorders

Eating Disorders: Anorexia Nervosa and Bulimia

Anorexia Nervosa
Serious disorder usually seen with teenage girls and of *higher* socioeconomic background (moviestars, musicians trying to "look their best"). The girl has a misperception that she is overweight and has to diet by different ways like: self-induced vomiting, extreme exercises, using diuretics and laxatives. This is done in order to "get rid of all that extra weight." In reality the person is starving their body and they have lost their form to appear cachectic. The girl maintains an appetite (in fact, they think about food all the time), but she will induce vomiting to avoid the weight gain. This causes psychological changes and hormonal problems leading to amennorhea. Anorexics often show bulimia (binge eating) and immediately thereafter, vomiting.

Diagnosis is made on the following:
The person's refusal to maintain body weight within 15% of norm. Fear of weight gain or becoming fat (actually, underweight).
Distorted self-image of body (they look in the mirror and say they are fat; actually, they are a "toothpick".)
Missing three *consecutive* menstrual periods. (Amenorrhea)

Other findings:
Loss of libido, constipation or diarrhea with laxatives, dry skin, loss of hair of the head, lanugo hairs on face/arms/legs (this is the "blond baby hair").
Orange-coloring or pigmentation of the palms and soles (eating massive amounts of carrots; beta-carotene);
Vomiting and dental problems (from the stomach acid dissolving the teeth–enamel erosion) and *alkalosis* (from the loss of acid). The vomiting and laxative abuse can cause electrolyte imbalances and serious cardiac arrhythmias (hypokalemia; $K+$), and tetany (hypocalcemia; $Ca++$) (also see hyponatremia / hypochloremia and alkalosis).

Anorexia Nervosa (continued)
Acrocyanosis— circulatory problem of hands and feet (they are sweaty/clammy/cold/blue). Raynaud's phenomenon (another circulatory problem where the fingers/toes become *pale* and *painful* when the person goes out in cold temp.).
The hormone imbalances and other behavioral problems cause an increase in self-starvation and suicide.
Eating disorders, like anorexia nervosa are associated with OCD (it is an *obsessive* or *compulsion* to act in the way that they do).

Bulimia Nervosa
A disorder of *binge eating* that is found in anorexia nervosa and other disorders). Bulimics have uncontrolled *binge eating*. Then, they self-induce vomiting, and other *extreme* dieting or exercise. This is done to avoid weight gain. Additional diagnostic criteria: at least 2 bingeing episodes a week (for at least 3 months).

Bulimia usually occurs between 20 and 30 years of age.

These patients are usually *over*weight and may have other problems. Depression, personality disorders, alcohol and other abuse problems are common.

Serotonin systems regulate appetite. 5-HT *agonists increase* food consumption and weight gain. Therefore, this is probably a disorder of *hyper*serotonin.

13
Sleep Disorders

Sleep Disorders
Excessive *daytime* sleepiness syndromes include: Narcolepsy, Sleep apnea (more in the elderly). Insomnias (inability to sleep) and Parasomnias (body rocking, somnambulism, night terrors). Environmental influences like alcohol) disrupt sleep, and subsequently affect the other body systems.

Sleep apnea is the cessation of breathing. It is common with snoring individuals who have a partially obstructed oropharynx. The loss of oxygen can last for long intervals (sometimes over 10 seconds) and the blood CO_2 level increases, leading to hyperventilation. *Obesity* and *alcohol* are aggravators of this condition. Problems like: hypertension, heart disease, respiratory infections, daytime drowsiness, and irritability. The treatment includes: discontinuing alcohol and other drugs, nasal continuous positive airway pressure (CPAP), and surgical reduction of the uvula-soft palate.

Narcolepsy
Sudden sleep attacks in the middle of normal activity. The following are part of narcolepsy:
> Excessive daytime sleepiness,
> Sudden sleep attacks,
> Cataplexy,
> Morning sleep paralysis,
> Terrible dreams.

Narcolepsy has been associated with heredity. Problems with rapid eye movement (REM) sleep, with shortened latency period between sleep and REM onsets. They also have *cataplexy* which is the sudden loss of muscle tone. The treatment includes antidepressants and *stimulants*. Narcolepsy is a serious disorder because of the problems associated with the lost attention (the student will do poorly, because she is having episodes of sleep). Other problems include an increase in accidents from automatically sleeping on the wheel or other location.

Sleep Disorders (continued)

Parasomnias

Sleep behaviors that are similar to those behaviors in the wakeful hours. For example, *Somnambulism* (otherwise known as sleepwalking) happens in the first hours of *deep* sleep and in other *non*-REM sleep stages. The person has an amnesia affect, and has no memory of sleepwalking. It can be injurious if the person walks out onto a stairway and falls, or hits objects, etc. *Jactacio nocturnus* or body rocking/head banging are repetitive movements of rocking or hitting the forehead against the bed or headboard (this can last for up to hours). *Pavor nocturnus* (or night terror) is different from a nightmare because the person does not recall any bad dream. Instead, the child with night terrors experiences a sudden burst of screaming and is uncontrollable. The child suddenly sits up in bed, frightened, and screaming. This lasts a couple of minutes, and then he goes back to sleep. The person must avoid injury (keep the bed clear of sharp objects; lock doors), administration of *benzodiazepines* for sedation.

Insomnia is a common symptom from stress, or other environmental influences, depression, and anxiety. Insomnia can also be a symptom of *restless leg syndrome* (where the legs make quick movements during sleep). Treatment includes: decreasing the stressors, and drug therapy like Bromocriptine or Clonazepam (sedative-hypnotics).

14
Adjustment & Personality Disorders

Adjustment Disorders
A stressful situation causes sudden onset of symptoms, but the symptoms resolve within 6 months. This is seen in young adults, and can be considered a diagnosis of *exclusion*. The problem is that it can get out of hand and become a more severe problem like drug abuse or psychosis.

Personality Disorders
Disordered behavior that is fixed and inflexible to other real events; a person's own way of dealing with situations that is maladaptive and affects others. Different personalities that become serious problems affecting work, school, and family life. They are usually distrusting, rejecting, and find blame in others. Often, having great difficulty with stressful situations. Histrionic and narcissistic personalities are mostly found in *women*. Antisocial personality is mostly found in men. Many of the features of the actual disorders are present in personality disorders for: paranoid, schizoid, schizotypal, antisocial, borderline, histrionic, narcissistic, avoidant, dependent, and obsessive-compulsive *personality* disorders.

An illness may appear with deviant behavior, and signifies a pathology. Personality develops early in life and stays reasonably *constant* with time. This characteristics, habits, and other behaviors form from interaction. The interaction brings out the biologic (genes) and the environmental (social/cultural) influences. Deviations in personality may arise from brain pathology or even body type, neurochemical and psychophysiologic changes.

Antisocial personality disorder
Difficult behavior, going against social norms. Think of the antisocial personality disorder patient when the following are present: impulsivity, hot temper, excitable, *high* novelty seeking, *low* harm avoidance (takes risks), and *low* reward dependence (these patients are insensitive and deceptive). This is considered a sociopathy. Poor > Rich. Usually this is found in criminals and first seen in deviant behavior before teen age. The majority of individuals with antisocial personality disorder are *men*.

Personality Disorders
Antisocial personality disorder (continued)
Associated behaviors (majority are antisocial): fire setting, runaways, deceitfulness, animal cruelty, drug and alcohol abuse, fighting, trouble with school, abusive, foul language, lying, arrests, early age sexual intercourse, prostitution, attention deficit hyperactivity disorder, homicide, accidents, gang membership, and *tattoos*. There is NO pill to treat this, just behavioral control techniques.

Histrionic personality disorder
Excessive emotional problems and affecting the relationships with others, they are seeking attention. The following are present: *high* novelty seeking and reward dependence, and *low* harm avoidance. Histrionic personality disorders are usually seen in *women*.

Narcissistic personality disorder
This person shows a grandiose sense of self-importance with no limit to brilliance, beauty, and other self-admirations. Think of this as a histrionic personality with an incredible ego. (Everything in the world should be about the person.) They have intense emotions, they have *high* novelty seeking and reward dependence, and *low* harm avoidance.

Borderline personality disorder
Impulsive and self-damaging (overspend, hypersexual, abusive), and labile mood, intense anger and lack of control, with recurrent suicidal thoughts. These persons are instable, have a difficult self-image and are impulsive. This is a mild mood disorder with some treatment from lithium, MAOIs, and carbamazepine.

Avoidant personality disorder
Socially inhibited, with negative feelings and unwillingness to become involved because of fear of rejection or criticism. They rarely take risks or get involved in new endeavors, because they are "embarrassed".

Dependent personality disorder
A continuously "dependent" person who needs to be taken care of continuously. They become submissive (even doing things that would be considered offensive) and they latch on to a person for their support. They have problems with doing their own things, because of loss of self-confidence.

Personality Disorders (continued)

Obsessive-Compulsive personality disorder
Person is preoccupied with perfectionism and order. They are "control wizzards" and must abide by the rules. Often never finishing projects because their own standards are too high or the point of the project was lost.

Schizoid personality disorder
Introverted, emotionally cold (emotional blunting), and the person is caught up with his own thoughts. They are daydreamers and fear becoming close with others. There is an increased family history of schizophrenia in relatives. Behaviors showing similar *positive* symptoms like delusions, illusions, thought disorder, speech problems and other problems. BUT, these persons are NOT psychotic. Remember, there are NO real lab exams. Treatment includes low doses of neuroleptics and being taught to discontinue behaviors.

Schizotypal personality disorder
These people are "odd" and communicate as if they are schizophrenic, but they are not. They have paranoid ideas, believe in magic, and their odd behavior is *worse* than in schizoid personality disorder.

Paranoid personality disorder
These people find suspicions behind any acts (usually acts of kindness from others), and cause conflicts with others. They are suspicious, envious and inflexible. Many times this is seen with disabled individuals or anyone feeling different than others.

Cloninger's Personality Classification
Novelty seeking– having an profound behavior with the need to search for ornate or new (novel) stimulation. Associated with *low* basal *Dopaminergic* activity.
Harm avoidance– avoiding punishment, or anything new that may cause problems. Associated with HIGH basal *Serotonergic* activity.
Reward dependence– reacting to rewards, and needing them to function.
Combination of **low** harm avoidance and reward dependence **plus high** novelty seeking = an anti-social personality,
Combination of **HIGH** harm avoidance and reward dependence **plus low** novelty seeking = passive-dependent and avoidance personalities.

Anxious and Fearful Personality Disorders

These personality disorders include:

Avoidant	*Low* novelty seeking, High harm avoidance, High reward dependence
Dependent	*Low* novelty seeking, High harm avoidance, High reward dependence
Passive-Aggressive	**High** novelty seeking, High harm avoidance, High reward dependence
Obsessive-Compulsive	*Low* novelty seeking, High harm avoidance, **Low** reward dependence

Low *novelty seekers* are: frugal, orderly, and regimented; or quiet, satisfied with life as it is, and reserved.

High *harm avoidance:* these people are very shy and inhibited; or they are always worried, cautious, and pessimistic.

Treatment includes: education, decreasing the stress, and counseling.

15
Neuropsychiatry Highlights

The Psychiatric Interview
In a diagnostic interview, the examiner collects information by asking questions, and observing the patient and the responses. A few affective techniques for increasing the patient's confidence in the examiner and developing a proper diagnosis:
Showing concern, empathy, interest, competence, and respect for the patient. Making observations and phrasing questions in an appropriate manner, focusing on certain topics, using information like the history from the patient and others (like family members), and a proper physical examination. The mental status examination begins immediately during the interview and continues by interacting with the patient. The interview may acquire information that will be very helpful in the diagnosis.

Deductive data is collected by the examiner's questioning based on knowledge. *Inductive* data is collected by using experience to ask questions, making observations and tests specific to the history given (this will "induce" the information collected).

Inductive questions to obtain a history include:
   What brings you here today?
   How many times has this happened?
   Have you ever been to a psychiatrist before?
   Is there any alcoholism or has anyone attempted suicide in your family?
   Do you have any medical problems?
   When you were a child, did you have problems with school?
   What kind of stress have you had with work or at home?
These questions will be very important in attaining information. They relate to the present problems, past history, family history, and social history. The mental status examination is an important part of the examiner's interview process, let us review it here...

Mental status examination (MSE)

The observations and tests in the MSE will highlight a possible psychopathology by bringing significance to the following areas of consciousness:

Arousal – Does the patient maintain attention?
Psychomotor activity – Does the person coordinate his movements properly? Be aware of the speech, hands, and body movements.
Mood – Does the patient show emotions?
Memory – Can the patient recall things?
Thought processing and content – Can the patient interpret things, and what exactly is he thinking about?

Administer tests. By correctly performing tests, the examiner may elicit a response (possibly inferring a psychopathology) that was not demonstrated during the observed examination.

Observation	Irregularities:
Appearance	Check for illness, inappropriate dress, and poor grooming.
Attention and arousal	Hyperalert, lethargic, stuporous, or comatose. Ability of patient to be attentive, lack of focus, difficulty with questions and requested tasks.
Psychomotor activity	Look for movement quantity and quality; whether the movements are increased or decreased, coordination problems, handshake and speech problems.
Speech	Slurred, pressured, inadequate speech relates to psychomotor function. Incoherent thought processing. Vocabulary deficits or superior – intelligence.
Affect	Facial expressions, voice and fine motor movements; observe the quality (inappropriate), intensity (constricted) and range (blunted, labile). The affect shows changes of psychomotor activity through these expressions.

Observation	Irregularities:
Mood	Euphoric or increased, irritable, depressed, neutral, anxious. Often in facial expression (i.e., omega sign in depressed patient; Ω -shape between brows on forehead; considered from the facial expression and bringing eyebrows together causing wrinkles in the lower forehead)
Memory	School and past history is relevant Immediate, recent, and long-term memory. Tests: Digit span (memorize and repeat 1,5,3,2,6) = immediate memory. Orientation and remembering objects if asked in a few (5) minutes = recent memory. Naming previous locations or presidents = Long-term memory.
Thought processes	Hallucinations, delusions, and thought associations. Describe the type and quality, and whether the hallucination is present (does the patient hear voices in his head?). Are there *persecutory* delusions; "Someone is after me, and he wants to kill me.", *grandiose* delusions; "I am Superman.", and/or delusions of *reference;* "The T.V. was talking about me.") Thought associations include loose or illogical ideas, tangential thought, rambling, and "flight of ideas". By testing with similarities and differences, you can recognize problems with abstract thinking and association.
Content	During the interview, the patient may make reference to unusual interests or problems. Suicide and homicide are examples.

Cognitive and Behavioral Neurologic Exam

Evaluate neurologic function and determine where the lesion is. Has the lesion affected the: brain stem, basal ganglia, cerebellum, motor and sensory nerves and tracts? These are locations of language processing, memory, and motor-spatial orientation. Patients may have impaired cognition. For example, schizophrenics (over half) and many bipolar patients have cognitive loss. In schizophrenics, the damage is diffuse and chronic with emotional blunting. In bipolar patients, it is frontal and visual-spatial. What is the level of consciousness? Is there diffuse impairment? How about cognitive function? And how do you interpret the results?

First, assess the level of consciousness:
Stupor, decreased consciousness, or full alertness.

Stupor

Associated with: catatonia, depression, mania, epilepsy, severe intoxication, and delirium. Giving I.V. *sodium amobarbital* will temporarily clear stupor for a patient speak and move, or eat. The *sodium amytal interview* helps the doctor to evaluate a patient.

Cognitive Function

Level of consciousness is assessed with orientation to person, place, and time. *Screening tests,* like the Mini-Mental Status exam, are done. Scores less than 24 increases the likelihood of coarse brain disease, and 20 or less indicates diffuse impairment. As a general rule, no tests are very sensitive; and as a result, do not rule out coarse brain disease.

Mini-Mental Status exam tests language function (five items) but does not test for abilities like: thinking, visual memory, or interhemisphere transfer. Therefore, must do further testing to assess cognitive function. It is useful for examining coarse brain disease. Is the patient saying things that are odd or broad, and therefore you test thinking and language. Talk of past happenings are out of sequence, and you test memory.

Motor Functions

Motor behavior is assessed by performing extrapyramidal, cerebellar, frontal, parietal lobe motor tests. Soft neurologic signs demonstrate brain dysfunction and are difficult to localize the problem; this is why they are called "soft" signs (see below). These soft signs are found in the majority of psychotic patients.

Soft neurologic signs:
Structural, Functional, and behavioral signs.
Look for asymmetry of face, scars, discoloration, enlarged hands, space in between fingers, etc. Sensory examination, reflexes, errors of language, speech, posturing, coordination and movement disorders.

Adventitious motor overflow
The appearance of choreiform movements when a patient is asked to hold both arms straight out. Involuntary hand movements, not agitation nor an anxious mood.

Motor impersistence or motor weakness
Can the patient keep a motor action. Consider a frontal lobe problem. Weakness of the upper extremity (with closed eyes) consider lesion in the *contralateral* parietal lobe.

Echopraxia
When the patient copies what the examiner is doing, even though he is told not to. Mimics the doctor. (i.e., the examiner moves his arm to a position for awhile, and tells the patient not to do "this". or "When I touch my nose, you touch your chin." If the patient touches his nose, then it is echopraxia. It is NOT *dominant* parietal dysfunction as in left-right disorientation. This is a "soft sign".

Gegenhalten
The patient forces *equal and opposite resistance* to anything the examiner does (even told not to resist).

Motor behavior occurs through the frontal lobe. In perseveration or the unnecessary repetition. Frontal lobe abnormalities: test constructional praxis by drawing a Greek cross. In perseveration, the person has a problem with starting the task. In *motor inertia,* the person has a tough time beginning a motor task, and then has a problem with stopping the task.

Motor sequencing
The patient taps a surface in a sequence by switching with the side of the fist, the outside of the hand, and then the palm.

Stimulus-bound motor behavior
motor actions can be controlled despite the presence of conflicting or distracting stimuli. Echopraxia and Gegenhalten are *stimulus-bound* behaviors.

Handedness
Right-handed person, usually *dominant* for language in the *left* hemisphere. The dominant hemisphere processes anything *symbolic,* like language.
> 97% of people are Left-sided dominant or left *and* right.
> 3% have the dominant hemisphere in the right.
> 90% of people are right-handed or *dextral.* (about 99% are left-sided hemisphere dominant).
> 10% of people are left-handed or *sinistral.*

Test handedness (i.e., which hand is preferred for writing or throwing a ball) when testing the motor function of the patient.

Idiokinetic or ideo*motor* praxis
The ability to perform a request; from memory, with no clues or help. Is there a lesion or detachment between hemispheres? Since patients with interhemispheric disconnection have normal idiokinetic praxis with the "dominant hand" but abnormal on the less used hand. We test this nonpreferred hand first. The patient is asked to show how to use a key with the nonpreffered hand (usually the left hand; makes a turn). The results: we see a normal hand movement in the one hand (contralateral to the dominant hemisphere), and abnormal in the opposite hand.

Remember, the *normal* hand movement (usually the right side) is contralateral to the dominant (usually the left) hemisphere. And abnormal in the other hand. [If *dominant parietal* lobe dysfunction is present, then idiokinetic dyspraxia occurs with *both* hands.]

Kinesthetic praxis
Being able to imitate certain hand *movements.* Dyspraxia occurs if the person cannot do this. There is a problem in the *parietal* lobe **contra**lateral to the hand that is tested.

Constructional praxis
Copying the outline of a Greek cross or other object on a blank piece of paper will show constructional praxia. If the object is drawn wrong, it is constructional **dys**praxia. Consider the location of the problem. If a drawing by the *preferred* hand is wrong, and the drawing with the other is correct, this means there is a problem with *interhemispheric disconnection.* If both drawings are incorrect, the problem is probably in the **non**dominant *parietal* area.

Remember, verbal reasoning occurs with the dominant hemisphere, and has nondominant parietal lobe function.

Dressing praxis

The ability to dress oneself or remove clothing with no assistance. Dressing *dys*praxia would signify a problem in the **non**dominant *parietal* area.

Language

Using symbols to communicate by speech, writing, or other form to bring understanding. The *dominant* hemisphere controls language. The *non*dominant hemisphere adds the creative gesturing (i.e., prosody).

Speech

Speech, or using words, originates from the parasylvian areas of: the temporal, frontal, and parietal lobes (in the dominant hemisphere). Speech *affect* originates in the *non*dominant hemisphere. Dominant hemisphere areas include: Broca's area, Wernicke's area, the arcuate fasciculus connecting Broca's to Wernicke's area, the temporal lobe, the supramarginal gyrus of the parietal lobe, and the motor cortex. Broca's area: involved in speech *fluency*. Broca's *aphasia* is a problem with speech fluency. This is also seen with frontal lobe problems and schizophrenia.

Nonfluent aphasias

Broca's Aphasia

Damage to the postero-inferior region of the *left frontal* lobe area (inferior frontal gyrus) results in Broca's aphasia. Patients with Broca's aphasia *understand* spoken language, but can**not** *express* themselves fluently or may be mute (impaired fluency of speech). They can't say what they want to say. They speak like a telegram (telegraphic speech: "bring tomorrow book" leaving out the connecting words). They are often dysarthric, and have a hard time with words and mispronounced syllables (i.e., "Bess estape" for "Best escape").

If a person has problems repeating entire sentences, then consider a problem more posterior. Look for decoding and phonemic expression problems. How much brain damage has occurred?

Look for:	Problems with:
Extremities (contralateral)	Weakness or paralysis
Dysgraphia	Handwriting usually problems on ipsilateral side).
Idiokinetic dyspraxia	The ipsilateral hand
Buccolingual dyspraxia	Facial and tongue movements: like blowing out a match, or whistling.

Lesions cause problems with the transfer of information from the left to the right premotor area and motor cortex resulting in aphasias.

> ***Trans*cortical *motor* aphasia** occurs from an injured frontal lobe Broca's area, in the dominant hemisphere; usually from *middle* cerebral artery occlusion. Speech is difficult and shortened, but the person can listen and understand (auditory comprehension), and can repeat sentences.
>
> ***Global* aphasia**: problems with *all* parts of speech; problems with hearing (comprehension), reading, and writing. This happens with an occluded *middle* cerebral artery.

Fluent Aphasias

Fluent speech, but is it understandable? Are the words being used correctly? Does the person comprehend what is being said? Fluent, nonunderstandable speech with poor comprehension suggests

> ### Wernicke's aphasia
> Speech that is difficult to understand, and the person has poor comprehension of someone else's speech. The lesion is located at *Wernicke's* area, at the *posterior* third of the *superior* temporal gyrus. This person will have the so-called "fluent" speech and have difficulty repeating things. Jargon speech = *driveling.* Everything about the speech is normal, but the *content* is meaningless. The person sounds like he is saying something, but it is just a bunch of words flowing with little meaning. Writing can also be aphasic.
>
> ### Conduction aphasia
> Similar to Wernicke's aphasia (they have repetition problems), but *normal* comprehension. Conduction aphasia patients have problems with word finding and with reading aloud. They make phonemic paraphasic errors. The lesion involves the *arcuate fasciculus* by the *dominant parietal* lobe.
>
> ### Transcortical sensory aphasia
> Also similar to Wernicke's aphasia (but repetition is normal). They can repeat difficult sentences, but have no clue as to what they are saying. Problems with reading and auditory comprehension. The lesion also involves the *angular gyrus* in the *dominant parietal* lobe.
>
> ### Thalamic aphasia
> The lesion is located near the *dominant thalamus.* Speech is *fluent* and the repetition is *normal.* Problems with comprehension can occur.

Thalamic aphasia (continued)
Problems: paraphasia, reading aloud, writing, and dysnomia or anomia (difficulty or inability to *name* objects). The lesions are in: the *left basal ganglia* (remember the "head of the caudate" during neuro lab; lesions in this area can cause *thalamic* aphasia).

Deciding on what type of aphasia
Normal repetition, but jargon speech suggests *conduction* aphasia (see the previous subsection).

Ask the patient to *name* objects (show him a watch, a shoe lace, or other object). Then, ask the patient to *point to* an object that you name. Problems suggest *thalamic* aphasia.

Repetition problems in Broca's and Wernicke's aphasias. Test for repetition problems, by asking the patient to repeat "difficult" phrases, like "Philadelphia cheese," "Minnesota mining," and difficult sentences like "No if's, and's, or but's." or "We moved where he was when she was there."

Dyslexia
Problems with reading and writing. This is considered one of the leading learning disabilities and if the person cannot read/write it is **a**lexia. Sometimes, *silent* reading comprehension is normal. The patient might not be able to read aloud. Ask the patient to read a list of words and sentences. The lesion is usually in the *arcuate fasciculus,* and there is a problem with not being able to connect Wernicke's area with Broca's area. If the person writes, but can't read, then there is a disconnection between the *occipital lobes* and *Wernicke's area.*

Wernicke's Aphasia	Broca's Aphasia
Fluent speech	Usually from *middle* cerebral
Jargon speech = *driveling*	
	Speech is difficult and shortened, but the person can listen and understand (auditory comprehension), and can repeat sentences.
Poor comprehension of speech	
Meaningless content	
May have Writing Aphasia	May have Writing Aphasia
Repetition problems	
	May be caused by *middle* cerebral artery occlusion.

Prosody and Gesturing
Non-dominant hemisphere language functions. If the dominant hemisphere is normal (has normal comprehension), but there is a lesion in the *non*dominant hemisphere have problems with range, accentuation, and melody of voice, gesturing, and understanding emotions of others in their speech. Evaluate prosody and gesturing by checking for speech changes in range and modulation. *Expressive* prosody–when the patient repeats a sentence that is emotionally neutral like "The television was turned on." Then, asking the patient to *involve emotions* in the sentence to make it sound and appear *sad and then angry.* *Receptive* prosody–stand behind the patient and assess only the *tone* of voice. Request which emotion (sad, angry, happy, or neutral) is in the sentence (say the sentence in voices with these emotions).

In *anterior* or frontal prosodic disturbance, the patient has problems with displaying in speech his emotions or gestures. In *posterior* or temporal prosodic disturbance, the patient has problems with comprehension prosody and gesturing of other people.

Thinking
Assess: the judgment, problem-solving skills, comprehension, concept formation, and reasoning.

Problem Solving
Assess: judgment and problem-solving skills, do longer math problems. Dyscalculia or acalculia = problems with math calculations or not being able to do mathematics. Seen with *dominant* hemisphere and parietal lobe problems.

Reasoning
Can the patient figure out what is not logical about a particular statement. And reasoning by looking at a series of pictures that have some senseless part in the picture (i.e., a picture of a house with no door).

Memory
There are five stages of memory

Stage 1	Primary sensory cortex receives input. (Cannot test)
Stage 2	(Cannot test)
Stage 3	Concentration. *Short-term* memory or *working* memory is forgotten within half a minute if it does not get stored further. Digit Span = Testing concentration and attention by reading a series of numbers (up to 7 number) and asking to repeat them forward and backward.
Stage 4	Transferring into memory by repeating or using mnemonics to rehearse information. Using visual or sounds (music) to remember. Test by showing items and asking to copy them the same size. Then, removing the shapes and asking to immediately recall the items. (at least 5 must be correctly drawn)
Stage 5	*Long-term* memory. Memory lasting longer than half an hour for as long as a lifetime. Storage sites: Secondary and Tertiary cortical locations of brain. *Autobiographical* memory – details and events in life are recalled.

Visual **memory**
A person has to keep attention and concentrate to remember. In order to memorize something visually, there needs to be connections between visual, language, and memory systems. This allows a person to see, read, and comprehend something. The *corpus callosum* allows bimanual tasks (without watching hands, like playing an instrument without looking at the guitar). When we learn something very well, it is part of the *dominant* frontal lobe function, and no longer the corpus callosum.

Visual-Spatial function
Recognizing visual and auditory or *non*verbal patterns, and spatial relationships.
Topographic orientation: problems finding the way around once-familiar areas.
Spatial recognition: left-right orientation, problems with not taking care of the *left* side of the body; the *left* side is neglected. This is seen with *non*dominant hemisphere problems. The *right* side is neglected in *left* frontal lobe lesions. Test the left and right side by doing left / right spatial tests (i.e., by crossing a set of slashes with a pencil). If the person crosses the left side, but has *right*-side neglect, then he most likely has a *left* frontal lobe lesion (see below).

X   X   X   X   /   /   /   /

X   X   X   X   /   /   /   /

Anosognosia = **not** recognizing an illness as a medical problem.
    Babinski's Agnosia: seen with patients who have paralysis or hemiparalysis and they try to walk even though they cannot (they can have an accident while getting out of bed).
    Anton's Syndrome: when a blind person thinks he can see. This happens with *non*dominant hemisphere problems.

*Prosopa*gnosia (*not* being able to recognize=*a*gnosia, a once-familiar face=*prosopo*).

Capgras' Syndrome: when the person believes that a once-familiar person is now unfamiliar (i.e., a patient may have a delusion that his brother is an impostor). This is seen with *posterior non*dominant hemisphere problems.

Fregoli's Syndrome: When a person believes (has a delusion) that an unfamiliar person is actually a relative or someone he knows.

Doppelganger phenomenon: This is also seen with *posterior non*dominant hemisphere problems. When a person has a delusion that a duplicate person or place also is somewhere else. The person may believe that he has a twin.

Graphesthesia
Taking the patient's hand, you "print" a letter on the palms with an unopened pen with closed eyes. First test the left side; or the side *ipsi*lateral to the dominant hemisphere. Then, test the preferred hand. If there is graphesthesia only in the *non*preferred hand, then, suspect problems with the corpus callosum **or** the *contra*lateral *parietal* lobe. If there is graphesthesia in the preferred hand, then the problem is in the *dominant parietal* lobe (contralateral to the preferred hand).

Stereognosis
Placing an object in the patient's palms. As with graphesthesia, first test the left side; or the *ipsi*lateral side of the *non*dominant hemisphere. Astereognosis = problems with the *contra*lateral *parietal* lobe or corpus callosum. Then, test the preferred hand. If there is astereognosis only in the *non*preferred hand, then, suspect problems with the corpus callosum **or** the *contra*lateral *parietal* lobe. If there is astereognosis in the preferred hand only, then the problem is in the *dominant parietal* lobe (contralateral to the preferred hand).

Overall, **graphesthesia and stereognosis** test the *parietal* lobe *contra*lateral to the tested hand, and tests the connection between the left and right hemispheres (corpus callosum).

Review:
Reviewing the clinical interview and the mental status examination, you can decide if the patient has cognitive impairment in a lobe or brain area. Does the lesion affect the dominant (language expression, usually left hemisphere) or the *non*dominant (usually right) hemisphere? If the person is right-handed, then the *left* (dominant) hemisphere is for language function. The *right* (*non*dominant) hemisphere is for visual-spatial function. The communications between the two hemispheres (the corpus callosum) is for exactly that: *communicating information between the two hemispheres!* This allows communication from with the *opposite* hemisphere.

In general, there are NO routine lab tests, they only help in the diagnosis or in the treatment plan. (i.e., there are NO lab tests that are specific for the diagnosis of mania or schizophrenia, and you must combine lab findings with patient history and examination.) Patient behavior is the most sensitive test. Don't get confused with the MRI's, CT's and other tests; just use them to confirm or rule out your differential diagnoses.

Lab Test	Used in the Diagnosis of:
Electroencephalogram (**EEG**)- Microvolts measured from the scalp, measured by polygraph with leads. The reference electrodes are placed on the ears. Look at the *amplitude* (or voltage; Hz) and the *frequency* (or cycles/second; cps). Try to have the patient come in with a little sleep deprivation, and off medication. Artifacts are a big problem of an EEG and come from muscle movement in the jaw/scalp/eyes, etc. You may cause an *evoked potential* by stimulating the patient with visual flashes of light or electrical stimulation; which causes an electrical activity (potential).	Schizophrenia, Bipolar Manic-Depressives, Coarse Brain Disease
	EEG interpretation
	Brain activity: (0.5 - 35 cps)
	Δ Delta 0.5 - 3.5 cps (deep sleep)
	θ Theta 4 - 7 cps (sleepy person)
	α Alpha 7.5 - 12 cps (resting person, alert with closed eyes.)
	β Beta 12.5 - 35 cps (alert person, concentrating)
	Muscle activity: > 35 cps.
	Changes in:
	Amplitude- High in epilepsy and delirium. A flash of bright light can cause a spike. Low in Parkinson's dementia, Huntington's and Alzheimer's).
	Frequency- Slow if lesions (brain loss). Fast in hyperactivity, and delirium tremens.
	Waves- Spikes and sharp in epilepsy. Petit mal seizure will have a wave pattern of **3** per second.
	Watch these changes over time as well.
	Evoked potentials– used in Multiple sclerosis, see a *delayed* wave formation and abnormal waveforms. This is because of the demyelination.
	Prolonged interwave periods– from compression of axons by Brain tumors; usually in localized areas.
	Normal potentials in patients who are hysterical.

Lab Test	
Neuroimaging Computed Tomography (**CT**)	CT measures the x-ray beam as it goes through the brain. Slices are divided into cubes called *voxels*. This gives us the CT image.
Magnetic Resonance Imaging (**MRI**)	MRI is preferred over CT because of the better resolution, safety, and less artifacts. The magnet realigns Hydrogen protons. You can get coronal images and see more detailed basal ganglia, amygdala, and hippocampus. Used for: tumors, multiple sclerosis, and infarcts.
Cerebral Blood Flow Imaging Single-Photon Emission Computed Tomography (**SPECT**)	SPECT– Xenon 133 or Iodine 123 isotopes emit photons. *Cerebral blood flow reflects brain cell activity.* Blood flows to the working areas. (Therefore, it is NOT used for structural lesions.) Caffeine and nicotine decrease flow. Anxiety increases flow. Alzheimer's have a decrease in flow; in the *posterior temporo*parietal regions. Depression either have normal or decreased flow (in frontal area usually).
Positron Emission Tomography (**PET**) Positively charged electrons (positrons) attach to molecules in the brain. This allows you to study the brain's cell activity and the blood flow; used mainly in research and not much in clinical setting. Fluorodeoxyglucose (FDG) is the tracer. Creates 3-D images.	PET is used for: Alzheimer's disease – **decreased** *posterior* cerebral blood flow. Pick's disease – decreased frontotemporal flow. Schizophrenia, mania, depression– decreased frontal flow (*hypo*frontality). Multi-infarct dementia, alcoholics and withdrawal, Smokers and caffeine / barbiturate abusers– decreased flow various areas Huntington's disease– **increased** frontal and decreased parietal flow Stimulant abusers– increased flow Anxiety disorder– increased parahippocampal and basal ganglia flow

85

Lab Test	Used in the diagnosis of:
Venereal Disease Research Laboratory (**VDRL**)	Central Nervous System **Syphilis** (rare)
Thyroid function tests, STD, etc.	Systemic Disease from Medical etiology (Endocrine disorders, and behavioral changes) (Refer to Neurologist.)

Neuropsychological Testing
Testing for changes in brain structure, cognition, and processing of information. Batteries of tests include: Halstead-Reitan, Luria-Nebraska, and the Wechlser Adult Intelligence Scale (WAIS- for intelligence).

Clear or Altered Consciousness
Sensorium: clear or altered
Cognitive impairment: diffuse or focal
Onset of the disorder: < 40 years old,
                        41 - 65, or
                        > 66 years old.

Establish a differential diagnosis (what may cause the problem?).

Possible Diagnosis	**Test used to confirm:**
Delirium	EEG- abnormality with *high*-voltage slow waves.
Drug-induced intoxication	Blood and urine screen for drugs.
Delirium tremens	EEG- abnormality with *low*-voltage fast waves. Problems with cognition.
Endocrine disorders	Thyroid function tests- abnormal. Etc.
Wernicke's Encephalopathy	Nystagmus, Ophthalmoplegia, Peripheral neuropathy.

Herpes Encephalitis	Temporal lobe- virus fairly specific for this area; EEG- sharp waves.
Coarse Brain Disease	Performance deficits, behavioral neuro exam abnormality. **EEG**- spikes or slow wave abnormalities. **MRI**- abnormality in structure does NOT identify coarse brain disease per say. (It does suggest brain disease if it is a **focal** lesion; NOT usually if it is a diffuse abnormality.) This is seen with Huntington's– atrophy of bilateral lenticulate areas.

Speech Irregularities	Characteristics:
Word Approximations	Using words or phrases without the accurate meaning.
Neologisms	Nonsense, made-up words.
Semantic Paraphasias	Real words that do not have a meaning for others.
Driveling Speech	Lost meaning of speech.
Tangential Speech	Changed point; Digression to another topic rapidly during a conversation.
Verbigeration	Continuously repeating meaningless words/phrases.
Perseveration	Repeating a previously correct response, but it is repeated again and in an inappropriate time.

Frontal Lobe Syndromes: Convexity and Orbitomedial Syndromes

Convexity Syndrome	**Orbitomedial Syndrome**
Lesions are located at the *lateral* surface of the *frontal* lobes. Presence of *negative* symptoms (i.e., emotionally unresponsive, *lack of* interest). Motor inertia– slow movements. Cataplexy– stay in the same position for a long time. (NO pill rolling like in Parkinson's). They walk alongside walls instead of taking the direct route in the middle of the walkway. If dominant hemisphere problems, then there is a problem with language and reasoning.	Problems with the *orbitomedial* areas in the *frontal* lobes. Presence of: euphoria, labile mood swings, and irritability. These people are very impulsive and go on "buying sprees", they are risk takers and make poor decisions. These uncontrollable desires are seen with their preoccupation with sex and other stimuli.

Temporal Lobe Syndrome
Remember, the temporal lobe functions in language and thought. Patients who have a stroke, a head injury, or an infection that affects this area (like viral herpes for instance) can have this syndrome. Also, vascular malformations and degenerative disease can cause these problems.

The patient may have: delusions, hallucinations (auditory and visual), mood changes, and fluent aphasia (temporo-parietal) and other language problems.

When the *dominant* (usually left side) temporal lobe is affected: euphoria, auditory hallucinations, formal thought disorder, delusions, and poor learning and retention are problems.

When the **non**dominant (right side) temporal lobe is affected: there are problems with irritability, dysphoria, depression, and receptive aprosodia (can't tell what feelings another person is expressing). They have problems with visuals, and have difficulty recognizing or recalling visual or auditory material.

Right Hemisphere Syndrome
This is usually the **non**dominant hemisphere. Lesions at the *posterior* location of the right hemisphere cause behavioral problems like: agnosia, denial, neglect, and aprosodia.

This is because they have problems with visual-spatial issues.

They are also irritable, anxious, and have disinhibited actions (like inappropriate sexual behavior).

Parietal Lobe Syndrome
Lesions in the **dominant** parietal lobe cause disorders of: language, like dyslexia, anomia, and aphasia, also problems with calculating, abstract thinking, and contralateral sensory problems like graphesthesia (unable to feel a letter written on the palm of the hand) and motor problems.
Gerstmann's syndrome: dysgraphia (problems writing), dyscalculia (problems with math), right-left disorientation, and finger agnosia (when cross fingers like prayer, they cannot tell which finger is which).

***

Lesions in the **non**dominant parietal lobe cause: anosognosia (denial of an illness), *left*-sided spatial neglect, problems with dressing, constructional problems and *contra*lateral sensory and motor losses.
Capgras' syndrome: having the idea (delusion) that a once-recognizable person like a relative is an impostor. They have the first-rank symptom, *experience of alienation* (certain parts of the body is not his).

Coarse Brain Syndromes
These syndromes will resemble mania, depression, schizophrenia, and even dysthymic disorder.
When trying to treat them, try the same medications as you would on the actual disorders. (see below)

Manic-like syndromes– try lithium or ECT.
Depressive-like syndromes– try ECT or tricyclic antidepressants.
Schizophrenia-like syndromes– try neuroleptics.
Dysthymic-like syndromes– try MAOI's or tricyclic antidepressants.

Characteristic Finding	Location of Lesion
Motor impersistence– can't keep eyes open, and Motor inertia– can't initiate movement	Frontal Lobe (anterior)
Problems with thinking and attention.	
Gegen**halt**en– opposing resistance; soft sign)	
Echopraxia– copies a movement when told not to.	
Perseveration– repeating words	
Neglect the **right** side of space	**Left** frontal lobe
Overlearn a bimanual task (tie shoelaces)	**Dominant** frontal lobe
***	
*Contra*lateral drifting of an extended handed	**Parietal Lobe**
Kinesthetic dyspraxia– can't copy hand movements.	*Contra*lateral parietal lobe

Characteristic Finding	Location of Lesion
Ideomotor Dyspraxias– simple motor tasks, like showing how to use scissors. Left-right disorientation. Disorders of language and calculation. Gerstmann's Syndrome– (Dysgraphia, left-right disorientation, and finger agnosia)	**Dominant** parietal lobe

***

Characteristic Finding	Location of Lesion
Constructional Dyspraxias– copy shapes, like a cross. Dressing problems. Left-spatial non-recognition– shaving on the right side, but not the left.	**Non**dominant parietal lobe
Capgras Syndrome (impostor, delusions, deny left space)	Posterior, nondominant parietal

Graphesthesia inability (printing letter on hand)
    On preferred hand
    On non-preferred hand
	Parietal Lobe:
	dominant hemisphere (ipsilateral)
	contralateral hemisphere

Speech– words and usage	Parasylvian areas of the frontal, temporal, and parietal lobes. In the *Dominant* hemisphere.
Speech– *affect* of speech	**Non**-dominant hemisphere.
Thalamic Aphasia (fluent) (problems reading, writing, and comprehension)	Dominant **Thalamus**
Problems reading aloud (can read and understand silently)	**Arcuate fasciculus** (between Wernicke's and Broca's area)

Condition	Associated with Neurotransmitter:
Mania	*Increased* **Dopamine (DA)**
Depression, Increased Food consumption, Bulimia	*Decreased* **Serotonin (5-HT)**
Satiety (satisfied, decreased food intake), Anorexia	*Increased* **Serotonin (5-HT)**

GABA (Gamma-aminobutyric acid)
This *inhibitory* neurotransmitter increases the *chloride* ion permeability of neurons. This *hyper*polarizes the axon and inhibits the excitation. GABA has a high affinity for benzodiazepines and this helps in treatment. The problem in patients with anxiety disorders is that they have a decreased number of GABA or benzodiazepine *receptors*.

Head Trauma Syndromes
Brain injury from accidents leaves victims with consequential disabilities. *Focal* deficits occur with the *penetrating* injuries. Close head injuries are the most common, and the causes of head injury include: automobile and sporting accidents (falls, and diving into shallow swimming pool). The patient can incur mild affects or brain syndromes, dementia, and seizures.

Post-Concussion Syndrome
Mild head injury and no real neuronal damage with slight loss of consciousness. Later, the person gets a headache, is hypersensitive to sound or light, has poor concentration, and is fatigued. Post-concussion syndromes resolve in a few days. If it persists, it can cause problems with the person's work or other life situations. The person may have problems with balance and vestibular problems. Any problems with cognition can use treatment similar to attention deficit disorder (amphetamines) or MAOI's. Propranolol is used with assaultive individuals.

Post-Traumatic Dementia
Severe closed head injury that has neuronal injury.

Post-Traumatic Thalamic Syndrome
When there is injury to the thalamus. No pain, and then pain. The person also has *tactile* hallucinations called *fornication* (like insects crawling on their body). Treatment includes: carbamazepine, tricyclic antidepressants, clonidine and beta-blockers.

Headaches
A pain or pressured *feeling* that has a sudden onset in the head. Causes of headaches include: eye problems, arthritis, dental problems, sinusitis, jaw problems, and hypertension. And yes, brain tumors can also increase intracranial pressure and can cause headaches.

> *Migraine* **headaches** are painful throbbing feelings in the head and can last for hours; they can also cause nausea and vomiting. They are usually **uni**lateral (on one side of the head). Vaso*constriction* from insults can cause a migraine. Increased in: young females (<30 years old, otherwise think of another medical problem) with a positive family history. Treatment can include: *Ergot*-preps, *sumatryptan,* and *propranolol.*

> *Tension* **headaches** are treated with aspirin or other analgesics. If the person has depression, then tricyclic antidepressants, MAOIs, or lithium (used in cluster headaches) is given.

Doing a Psychiatry Consultation
When receiving a request for a consultation, attend to the patient within 1 day if it is a routine consultation. If it is an emergency, then offer the physician the consultation within minutes. Talk with the patient's primary physician, then talk with the patient, and offer recommendations to both the physician and the patient. (Some doctors do NOT want the consultant to write orders on their patients, so ask the doctor if your recommendations should be followed with specific orders for the staff) Add extra history and possible drug interactions causing the findings. What specific treatments are recommended and if the patient needs additional psychiatric follow-up or may be discharged, etc.

Epilepsy

Seizure disorders can cause irregular behaviors. There are three types of seizure disorders: Generalized, Localized, and Mixed.
Generalized seizures
Petit mal, myoclonic, infantile spasms, tonic, clonic, tonic-clonic (grand mal), atonic, and akinetic seizures.
Localized seizures (partial epilepsy)
Simple– no loss of consciousness; but, motor and sensory symptoms
Complex– seizure attacks have disordered consciousness and behavioral problems.

Behavioral changes and epilepsy
The ictal state = time of seizure,
The *prodromal* period (hours to weeks before the seizure): Irritability and dysphoria.
The *post*ictal period (hours to days after the seizure).
The *inter*ictal period is less than 1 minute.

Temporal lobe epilepsy (TLE)
Most common type of psychosensory epilepsy, with a change in consciousness, and *oneiroid* or dreamlike states. The person has episodes of disorientation and irritability and unresponsive to stimulation (unless it is very profound). The person can have *automatisms* or repetitive behaviors (i.e., repeating sentences), crying, laughing, yelling, coughing, and other irregular behaviors.

Temporal lobe epilepsy (TLE) (continued)

Prior to the seizure (**pro**dromal):
- Intense changes in mood
- A feeling of impending doom and anxiety
- Problems with vision
- Oneiroid states or feeling of dreaminess
- Deja vu and jamais vu
- Visual, olfactory (smell) and gustatory (taste) hallucinations
- Autonomic Nervous System problems (i.e., heart palpitations, feeling cold, etc.)
- Gastrointestinal symptoms (i.e, abdominal pains "coming up into my head").

During a seizure (ictal), these can occur:
- The patient may be open-eyed, and stare in one direction without blinking.
- Cyanosis around the lips, and salivating
- Loss of posture
- Pupillary dilatation
- Sweating, tachycardia, and HTN (hypertension)
- Respiratory problems and apnea
- Urinary incontinence

After the seizure (**post**ictal):
- Usually have *amnesia* or forgetting that the event occurred
- Fatigue with sleepiness, confusion (absentminded), and maybe depression.
- Unusual sexual behaviors (like taking off clothes in public without realizing it).
- Behaviors can last from a few minutes to many hours or days.

Between seizures (**inter**ictal):
- The person may be a slow thinker
- The person may dwell on things almost obsessively
- Emotionally labile (they can show incredible anger, and then follow it with very loving attitudes)
- Some patients may have intellectual deterioration with progressive dementia (as a result of long-term phenytoin or primidone therapy)

Between seizures (**inter**ictal continued):
- Psychosis may occur, with a schizophrenia-like pattern
  But, the person has an affect that can show feelings (NOT emotionally blunted like schizophrenics). They also maintain their overall personality, and have more normal social-vocational-educational lives. The psychotic characteristics include: delusions, hallucinations (usually auditory or visual), catatonia, mood changes, and fear. We can also see: insomnia, loss of interest and appetite, and irritability.
- They can form: delusions of grandeur, hallucinations, and catatonia.

Pseudoseizures
"Fake seizures" that happen after a stressful event. The EEG is normal. These patients display the *symptoms* of true seizures. They have a change in consciousness, possible memory loss, and can be unresponsive to stimuli. Tongue biting and injury, loss of reflexes (i.e., corneal reflex), incontinence, and drowsiness after the "seizure" can be seen. Test if can induce a seizure by administering under controlled environment (i.e., EEG, protective setting, etc.): IV **saline**.

Treatment for Seizures
Carbamazepine is the *drug* of choice, and **ECT** can be the *treatment* of choice. An anticonvulsant drug is prescribed, and the patient's seizures are recorded. There are checks on the serum drug levels, and follow-up appointments. (Combination of two drugs is given if the one drug is not effective, but the BEST is to use only ONE drug.) Medication is given until the patient has no attacks for 2 to 4 years. People are usually not given longer-term therapy. Neuroleptics can be rapidly withdrawn; but *anticonvulsants* require a longer withdrawal time because discontinuing the drug abruptly may *induce* a seizure. *Pseudo*seizures are really NOT epilepsy, and the seizure attacks need to be treated with alternative therapy like: hypnotherapy, and counseling; otherwise, Benzodiazepines.

Additional topics for review:

Form is different from **thought content** of speech.

Constricted mood shows *one* mood (either depressed or sad).

Mood = the *content* of *affect* = range/intensity/stability (quantitative).

Aphasia
The inability to process language appropriately. Impaired *dominant* lobe functioning that results in impaired speech, writing, language, and other communication abilities.

Apraxia
The inability to do *voluntary* movements and complex motor activities. Inability to use an object properly.

Agnosia
The inability to recognize or accurately identify something.

Memory Problems
Problems with forgetfulness, concentration and distractibility. To assess the patient, take a good history and then proceed with *cognitive testing*. Think of the related disorders causing memory problems: depression or mania, alcohol or drugs, anxiety disorders, adjustment disorders, and even with "normal" people. can be an early sign of dementia.

Frontal lobe lesions can cause the following symptoms: confabulation and perseveration, and loss of inhibition (give the incorrect answer with no logic).

16
Psychopharmacology & Other Treatments

Common Medications in Psychiatry

Neuroleptics
Antipsychotic medications. (i.e., Chlorpromazine) They are highly lipo*philic*, and block dopamine (DA) thus, affecting the pathways:
Nigrostriatal system causing neuroleptic extrapyramidal side effects and is causally unrelated to the antipsychotic activity of the neuroleptics.
Block the tuberoinfundibular system causing hormonal changes like hyper***prolactin****emia* (which manifests as a pseudo-pregnancy with lactation)
Act as antipsychotics because they block the dopamine in the limbic system.

Alpha-adrenergic blockade with some neuroleptics causes a **hypo**tensive effect.
Anticholinergic effects (i.e., thioridazine) and *antihistamine* and *antiserotonin effects*.
They also have *potentiation* of depressants like alcohol and barbiturates.
Approximately 1 out of 7 patients on long-term neuroleptic treatment develop *tardive dyskinesia*. They have uncontrolled choreiform movements evenafter the medication is discontinued. The tardive dyskinesia appears as extrapyramidal side effects with tongue protrusion, lip smacking and other behaviors. All as a result of a midbrain biochemicalchange (too much dopamine in the basal ganglia or receptor sites). The treatment includes: Reserpine or physostigmine (But, NOT anti-parkinsonian agents). Therefore, only use these on seriously *psychotic* patients. Some items about neuroleptics that you should be aware of:

> Neuroleptics also cause *orthostatic **hypo**tension* (from blocking $\alpha 1$-adrenergic receptors).

> *Photosensitivity* occurs so keep the patient covered during the summer otherwise they will develop a very painful sunburn (may form papules) and wear sunglasses!

> *Neuroleptic malignant syndrome* and a malignant hyperthermia can cause death (to treat, give Bromocriptine, Dantrolene or ECT).

Neuroleptic Use (continued).
Chlorpromazine has been associated as a cause for *agranulocytosis* (SO check the *white* blood cell count; stay above 4,000 cells/cc).

Autonomic Nervous System side effects include: dry mouth, stuffy nose, blurred vision, constipation, and *paralytic ileus*.

Contraindications include: narrow-angle glaucoma, prostatic hypertrophy, prior reactions like agranulocytosis, breastfeeding and pregnancy (since neuroleptics are excreted in the mother's milk, and cross the placenta and enter the fetal brain).

Cyclic Antidepressants

These antidepressants get their potency and sedative properties from the side chains. They have either 1, 2, 3, or 4 ring structures (monocyclic...tricyclic, etc.). An example is *Fluoxetin* (Prozac), which is bicyclic. These can be absorbed by the G-I and they are metabolized by *demethylation* into a more lipophilic, active drug. Then, they are *hydroxylated* and *conjugated* to be excreted in the urine.

Side effects include: anticholmergic effects, with dry mouth, blurred vision, constipation, urinary retention, and a fine tremor. An overdose of cyclic antidepressants can cause *drug induced psychosis*, and *delirium*. If an overdose occurs, we give a *cholinesterase inhibitor* (a couple mg of Physostigmine I.V., repeated in 20 mins, and again in 30 mins).

Anticholinergic drug-induced delirium can be memorized by the common saying "mad as a hatter, red as a beet, dry as a bone, and blind as a bat."

[Do NOT administer tricyclics to patients with: Narrow-angle glaucoma and severe prostatic hypertrophy.

Monoamineoxidase Inhibitors (MAOI's)

These drugs are effective (usually in combination) for the treatment of: melancholia, anxiety disorders, dysthymia, and atypical depression. In combination with Lithium, MAOI's can help in the treatment of *bipolar affective disorder*.

Hydrazine derivatives are the most effective MAOI's. *Phenelzine* is an example. Non-hydrazines are similar to amphetamines. *Tranylcypromine* is an example drug; it is less effective.

MAOI's act by *inhibiting* the mitochondrial *enzymes* that *oxidize* the *monoamines*. The common monoamines are: serotonin (5-HT), norepinephrine (NE), and dopamine (DA).

Monoamineoxidase Inhibitors (MAOI's continued)
MAOI's are metabolized by the liver. Some individuals are *slow acetylators* (i.e., some Asians) who have a *slower* metabolism of the drug. This leads to a greater blood level. Thus, a gradual administration of the drug is necessary to avoid bad side effects; slowly increasing the dosage with time.

Hypertensive crisis can occur if foods with a high *tyramine* content are consumed (like cheese). The crisis consists of: hypertension, an intense headache, and a possible subarachnoid hemorrhage. We treat this crisis with: an α-adrenergic blocker like *Phentolamine*. If the patient notices the signs of a crisis coming, he should take a calcium-channel blocker, like *Nifedipine*, (taken sublingually) which has an α-adrenergic blocking effect to avoid the crisis.

[Do NOT give MAOI's with barbiturates. MAOI's potentiate CNS depressants like barbiturates.]

Fluoxetine (Prozac)
A serotonin (5-HT) reuptake inhibitor. This selective inhibition has a decreased number of anticholinergic effects (compared to TCA's which inhibit the uptake of all three: NE, DA, and 5-HT). This drug has a long half-life. It has been used successfully as an anti-depressant and in the treatment of obsessive-compulsive disorder.

Lithium
This is an interesting "drug", it is an alkali metal and is not organic (remember the chemistry table you learned in college and "carbons" in organic chemistry; Li has no carbons, it is by itself!). Many persons used to take baths in "natural springs", the lithium in the earth's crust and the water were "therapeutic" for many people and had a calming effect. Lithium is now the drug of choice in *bipolar affective disorder* and *mania*. It passively diffuses into cells and is NOT stored.

Lithium is used in unipolar (mania) and bipolar affective disorder (manic-depressive) because it also has an antidepressant effect. It is also used in treating: eating disorders (like anorexia nervosa and bulimia), drug abuse (usually the abuse is due to a mood disorder, and this drug helps in treating the mood disorder). The reason it is helpful in anorexia is because it causes some weight gain. Lithium has also been used for treating: headaches, PMS, OCD and anxiety disorders.

Lithium (continued)
Serum lithium levels should be taken to avoid toxicity. The signs of near toxicity include: fatigue, drowsiness, a fine tremor, nausea, polydypsia (increased thirst) and polyuria. This may need to decrease the dose, or add a P-blocker to offset effects. Take lithium with food. Toxicity usually occurs at levels > **2.0** mEq/l. *Toxicity* includes: vomiting or diarrhea, ataxia, slurred speech, a *coarse tremor*, lethargy, stupor, and even coma. This requires: discontinuance of the drug and supportive treatment. We force feed these patients with salty foods; there is NO drug to counteract the effects of Lithium toxicity, only hemodialysis. Therefore, try NOT to prescribe lithium to persons with renal problems.

Lithium has an anti-thyroid affect, and inhibits ADH. It does this by inhibiting the cAMP-adenyl cyclase, which affects the thyroid hormones (T3 and T4), and antidiuretic hormone (ADH). This causes polyuria. *Polyuria* is very common within the first couple of weeks of treatment, because sodium gets replaced by some of the Lithium until it reaches a steady state.

Lithium may be teratogenic, and is excreted in the breast milk. Therefore, mothers on lithium should NOT nurse their babies, instead feed them a bottled substitute.

Common, undesirable physical side effects include: *weight gain* and *acne*. By decreasing the dose, you may control these side effects.

NSAID's (like aspirin and indomethacin) can cause a *higher* serum lithium level. Therefore, the lithium dosage should be decreased. Other drugs increase the lithium *excretion*, like: osmotic diuretics, caffeine, and theophylline can *lower* serum lithium levels.

Anticonvulsants
Carbamazepine and valproic acid may be used to stabilize mood. They are metabolized by the liver and are scheduled throughout the day to maintain a therapeutic blood level.

Carbamazepine
Works as an anticonvulsant by acting on the sodium channels and benzodiazepine receptors. It is used for resistant types of mania and bipolar affective disorder.

Carbamazepine *decreases* haloperidol blood levels.

Anticonvulsants (continued)
Valproic acid
Acts as an anticonvulsant; GABA-agonist. It is used for acute mania and panic disorder. *Alopesia* (hair loss) is a undesirable side effect of this drug.

Discontinuation of both carbamazepine and valproic acid treatment should be gradual.

Anxiolytics
Cyclic antidepressants and MAOIs are used to treat anxiety disorders. Barbiturate and nonbarbiturate sedatives-hypnotics. Benzodiazepines are safer for their decreased abuse potential and wider safety margin in an overdose.

Benzodiazepine	Used in treating:
Benzodiazepines in general	Treatment of choice for acute **anxiety** states or **panic attacks.**
Triazolam, Temazepam, and Flurazepam	**Insomnia.** They have hypnotic effects and are used for bedtime sedation.
Benzodiazepines in general (Chlordiazepoxide or Diazepam)	Treatment of choice for **alcohol withdrawal** (the person has tremors, and is disoriented and restless)
Alprazolam	**Dysthymias**
Lorazepam	**Catatonia**

The absorption rates differ in benzodiazepines (Diazepam is *quickl*y absorbed; Oxazepam is *slowly* absorbed).

Commonly Used Benzodiazepines

Triazolam: *short*-acting,
Lorazepam: *intermediate*-acting,
Diazepam and Chlordiazepoxide: *long*-acting benzodiazepines.

Benzodiazepines are used for:
> Treating acute *anxiety* states,
> Bedtime sedation and hypnotic affects, and
> Drug of choice for alcohol withdrawal.

[Benzodiazepines enhance the GABA binding to its receptor site; increases the inhibitory effects.]

Sedatives

Barbiturates are the drugs for controlling agitated and violent persons. They are NOT more dangerous than neuroleptics. They have a rapid onset, and have *controllabl*e side effects. The sedation effects is more than neuroleptics. *Sodium amobarbital* is the drug of choice. *IV sodium amobarbital* can offer rapid sedation with little worry about respiratory depression.

A search for weapons must be part of the ER admission. Psychiatric patients are usually *NOT* violent. Their violent behavior can usually be *predicted*. For example, they usually display a behavior or history of: violent thoughts and intentions, they are jealous, have delusions and hallucinations, drug or alcohol *intoxication*, mania or depression, are suicidal, antisocial personality, fire-setters, own weapons, other family or gang violence. Look for tattoos, needle-tracks, agitation and pacing. If they appear threatening (angry and irritable, with pressured speech). Do they have some jealousy or revenge out for others? Any delusions?

Remember behavioral science: *previous actions can predict future behavior.* Therefore, violent criminals DO have an increased long-term risk for violent behavior.

The idea is to *prevent* this violence. Don't argue or go against an agitated and incapacitated patient. Comfort the patient, if this doesn't work, give sodium amobarbital or Haloperidol to sedate the patient (IM). Know where the hospital's panic button or emergency systems are.

If you can't *prevent* violence, then CONTROL it! Have a *psychiatric crisis team* ready to respond if there is a violent and physically uncontrollable patient. Say the command to "Stop" and put out your palm like a traffic cop. The person should then be restrained by the crisis team (usually the doctor and 3-4 others; one for each limb). The doctor should continuously try to "calm" the patient and direct the force to control the situation. Give a sedative and bring the patient to a secluded room. Restraints are placed on the extremities and strapped to the bed; the head is kept from harming (biting) the team members. Once he is sedated or calm then the restraints can come off and you can "work with" the patient.

Drug Dosage
It is important to give an adequate dose when prescribing psychoactive drugs and it is probably better to be on the upper end rather than the lower range for effectiveness.

Choose the *type* of preparation and the route of administration (drug absorption for the onset of action). *IV* or *IM* injection gives the fastest and largest blood level, then, *oral* tablets and timed-release capsules (filled with little doses of the drug).

Dose *scheduling* is also important, and the best scenario is a *single* daily dose because it increases compliance:
- Especially if it is administered at bedtime (sedative side-effects can be desirable at night, and unwanted in the daytime).
- At the privacy of home, there is no social problem of "being seen in a public place, taking drugs".
- Because it is easier to keep track of taking a medication one time per night.

Bioavailability is the amount of drug that circulates freely in the blood; it relates to how the drug becomes *available to the target organ* and in psychiatry this organ is the brain. It involves the drug's passage through the body and its resulting metabolism and excretion, the distribution into fatty tissue, the protein binding properties. The first-pass effect occurs as drugs "first pass" through (and are metabolized by) the *intestine* (usually slightly modified by the mucosa) and then the *liver* (through the portal circulation). **Lipo**philic drugs like the neuroleptics and tricyclic antidepressants are reabsorbed by the *enterohepatic cycle* (the liver). Demethylation, conjugation, and protein binding can occur.

Interactions with other drugs can occur. Alcohol and the nicotine of tobacco induce *liver* enzymes and therefore, need a larger dose of the drug to get a therapeutic blood level. The kidneys can play a role in the blood levels of Lithium (renal plasma flow). Although, the majority of drugs are bound to plasma *albumin*.

When the treatment does not work
Consider increasing the dose or prescribing a new drug. Decide if it was: not a good drug choice, misdiagnosed, inadequate dosage, or other issues (like poor compliance).

Electroconvulsive Therapy (ECT)

Notice: We will now discuss ECT as a treatment and its procedure. The following is a summary of the key events during the treatment, and should be used as a review only. As with all medications and procedures recommended in this book, we have simplified the content to a great extent. Never try these drugs or procedures without the full diagnostic, treatment, and procedure guidelines of other references. This is for review ONLY.

ECT is given with anesthesia and muscle relaxants; monitoring with CG and EEG, and other vital signs.

ECT is the most rapid treatment used as an antidepressant. Depression, psychomotor retardation, *early*-morning waking, and delusions are predictors of a favorable response to ECT. Hypochondriasis, anxiousness, and fear are predictors of an unfavorable response.

Manic patients who have failed to respond to medical treatments like lithium or neuroleptics, may respond to ECT treatment. A response is seen immediately, but requires up to 15 treatments to *treat* the illness.

Catatonia with stupor (mute, stupor, and catalepsy) also responds to ECT.

The ECT Procedure:
>To prepare the patient for ECT, a good history and physical examination is taken; the patient will be under general anesthesia and a medical screening with EKG, *chest* X-ray (NOT spine or head),, urinalysis, BS (fasting blood sugar), and BUN arc done. Obtain an *informed consent* from the patient or family/legal guardian. *Suicidal* patients who are a *danger* to themselves or other, an *emergency* ECT or involuntary ECT is allowed without the written informed consent (otherwise, get legal clearance).

>On the day of treatment, the patient should NOT eat or drink anything (NPO) because he may vomit and aspirate during treatment. You should remove anything that can cause injury to the patient (i.e., dentures, eyeglasses, jewelry). A mouth bite will offer protection for the teeth, tongue and mouth. Restrain the patient from having excessive leg and arm movements.

>*Atropine* or *Glycopyrolate* is given right before treatment to decrease the risk of a vagal response causing *brady*cardia, this also decreases the lung secretions.

The ECT Procedure (continued):
Methohexital (an ultra-short acting barbiturate) is the anesthetic given IV. The response to the anesthetic will take place after counting aloud to 50.

Then, *Succinylcholine* is given as the muscle relaxant. Muscle fasciculations will occur as the succinylcholine takes its role; affecting the face, upper extremities and finally the lower extremities. Once these have stopped, the patient is prepared for ECT.

Proper *Oxygenation* with positive-pressure is given for ventilation, until the patient is able to ventilate on his own. Carefully apply the electrodes on the scalp. **Bi**lateral ECT includes electrode placement on each side of the head. **Uni**lateral ECT includes electrode placement at the temporo-parietal area on one side of the head (the side of the **non**dominant hemisphere; usually the right-side). Unilateral ECT decreases the amount of memory loss and confusion.

Sinusoidal or alternating currents of electricity flow through the electrodes. These brief pulses stimulate the brain and *induce seizures*. These induced and controlled seizures are therapeutic. The side effects include: *temporary* disorientation and memory loss (*temporary* **retro**grade amnesia—for events before the treatment, and *permanent* **antero**grade amnesia—for events immediately after the treatment)- less with unilateral treatment.

Sedate the patient with *Diazepam*; you can also terminate any prolonged seizures (lasting > 3 mins.) with diazepam. *Pseudocholinesterase* is the enzyme that degrades succinylcholine, some patients may be deficient in this enzyme, and therefore require more assistance. Intubate the patient if respiration has not returned within 10 minutes.

[ECT has been challenged by many authorities, and the established risk : reward benefit over medications is not confirmed. Older patients may have a better *response* after ECT than younger patients. But, the risk of ECT may be substantial to warrant reconsideration since the patient will still need maintenance therapy with antidepressants, lithium, or anticonvulsants.]

The Elderly Patient
Since a large portion of the population in the upcoming years will be increasing in the number of elderly patients, and the body's physiology changes, and the onset of iatrogenic (physician-induced illnesses usually from drugs). By the year 2030, the elderly will constitute an estimated 20% of the population.

The most common illnesses include: mood disorders like depression, and coarse brain disease (dementia and delirium). Diseases cause cell death and changes in DNA. Aging or *senescence* causes a decline in *physiologic* function. Diseases and other illnesses like cerebral arteriosclerosis, multi-infarctions, heart disease, cancers, and dementias cause difficulty in the elderly. The elderly tend to be on multiple-drug treatments, and can develop drug toxicities. The body metabolizes and eliminates the drugs differently (lower liver– and kidney function–decreased renal clearance). Antacids have aluminum, magnesium, and calcium; these can *decrease* the absorption of certain medications like benzodiazepines and neuroleptics. Medication is the main cause of *delirium* in the elderly; due to dehydration, fever, decreased cardiac output, electrolyte imbalance, and hypoxia. Sexual dysfunction is a complaint.

Problem	Treatment of Choice in Elderly
Melancholia **Catatonia**	ECT or anti-depressants.
Mania	Lithium is the treatment of choice for all manic patients.
Dysthymia	Antidepressants, MAOIs, and psychotherapy, (same as in the younger patients, but a decrease in the dosage may be necessary)
Schizophrenia	Neuroleptics

This concludes our review of Psychiatry, re-read it a couple of times to put the concepts to memory. With this knowledge, you have the information to recall many of the psychiatric illnesses and their treatment. Good luck on your exams.

INDEX

Acetaldehyde dehydrogenase 32
Acrocyanosis 64
Activated charcoal 34
Acute mania 49
Adjustment Disorders 67
Affect 15, 16, 72
Agitation 12
Agnosia 98
Agoraphobia 54
Agranulocytosis 40
AIDS 35
Akathesia 14
Akinetic mutism syndrome 13
Alcohol 34
Alcohol Intoxication 8, 32, 33
Alcohol Withdrawal 33, 103
Alcoholic hallucinosis 33
Alcoholics Anonymous 32
Alcoholism 12, 32
Alpha-adrenergic blockade 99
Alprazolam 56, 103
Alzheimer's Disease 25, 26
Amnesia 59, 107
Amnestic Disorder 25
Amphetamines 34, 37, 46
Anafranil 22, 55
Androcur 62
Angel Dust 37
Anorexia 93
Anorexia Nervosa 63, 64
Anosognosia 82
Antabuse 32
Anti-motivational syndrome 36
Anticholinergic effects 99
Anticonvulsants 102, 103
Antidepressants 100
Antipsychotic medications 99
Antisocial 67
Antisocial personality disorder 11, 67, 68
Anton's Syndrome 82
Anxiety 12, 23
Anxiety disorders 53, 56
Anxiolytics 14, 34, 103
Aphasia 77, 78, 79, 98
Appearance 72
Appropriateness 16
Apraxia 98
Aprosodia 16
Arousal 72
Arylcyclohexylamines 36
Asperger's Disorder 24
Aspirin 27
Attention Deficit Hyperactivity Disorder 21
Autistic Disorder 21, 24
Automatic obedience 13
Automatisms 95
Autonomic Paroxysms 44
Avoidant 70
Avoidant personality disorder 68

Babinski's Agnosia 82
Basal Ganglia Disease Dementia 27
Behavior Therapy 56
Benzodiazepine 56, 66, 103, 104
Bereavement 51
Binge eating 64
Bioavailability 105
Bipolar affective disorder 8, 50, 100, 101
Blood alcohol level 32
Body dysmorphic disorder 58
Borderline personality disorder 67, 68
Brief Psychotic Disorder 41
Brief Reactive Psychosis 45
Briquet's syndrome 57
Broca's Aphasia 77, 79
Bromocriptine 46, 66, 99
Buccolingual dyspraxia 77
Bulimia Nervosa 63, 64

Caffeine 34
Cannabis 34, 36, 37, 46
Capgras Syndrome 82, 90, 92
Carbamazepine 44, 97, 102
Catalepsy 29
Catatonia 12, 29, 30, 103, 108
Catatonia type- Schizophrenia 42
Catecholamine hypothesis 50
Child Development 17
Chlordiazepoxide 53, 103
Chlorpromazine 40, 99, 100
Circumlocutory speech 11
Clomipramine 22, 55
Clonazepam 66
Cloninger's Personality Classification 69
Clozapine 40
Coarse Brain Syndromes 90
Cocaine 34, 35, 37, 46

Coffee 34
Cognitive Anxiety 53
Cognitive Function 74
Complete Auditory 45
Computed Tomography 85
Conduct Disorder 21
Conduction aphasia 78
Constructional Dyspraxias 92
Constructional praxis 76
Consultation 95
Content 73
Conversion disorder 57, S8
Convexity Syndrome 88
Cushing's disease 51
Cyclothymia 51
Cylert® 21
Cyproterone 62

Dantrolene 46, 99
Deductive data 71
Deja vu 44
Delirium 8, 12, 25, 26, 33, 86
Delirium Tremens 33, 86
Delusional Disorder 41, 42
Delusional mood 43
Delusions 8, 40, 43, 73
Dementia 8, 25, 26, 28
Dependency 31, 36
Dependent 70
Dependent personality disorder 68
Depersonalization 44
Depersonalization Disorder 59
Depression 8, 10, 12, 47, 93
Depressive pseudodementia 49
Derealization 44
Desipramine 35
Developmental Disorders 19
Developmental Milestones 17
Dexamethasone Suppression Test 49
Dexedrine® 21
Dextroamphetamine 21
Diazepam 33, 53, 103
Disorganized type- Schizophrenia 42
Dissociative Amnesia 59
Dissociative Anesthesia 35
Dissociative Disorders 59
Dissociative Fugue 59
Dissociative Identity Disorder 59
Disulfiram 32
Dopamine 93

Doppelganger phenomenon 82
Down's Syndrome 26
Downward drift 39
Dressing praxis 77
Driveling speech 11, 78, 87
Drug Abuse 34
Drug Dosage 105
Drug-induced abnormal movements 14
Drug-induced intoxication 86
Drug-induced Psychosis 46
DSM-IV™ manual 7, 9
Dysacousia 44
Dyscalculia 90
Dysgraphia 77, 90
Dyskinesias 15
Dyslexia 79
Dyspareunia 61
Dysphoria 47
Dyspraxias 92
Dysthyrnia 48, 103, 108
Dystonias 14

Eating Disorders 22, 63
Echolalia 30
Echopraxia 30, 75, 91
ECT 29, 40, 97, 106
ECT Procedure 106, 107
Ectomorph 12
EEG 84
Ego 18
Elderly Patient 108
Electroconvulsive Therapy (ECT) 106
Electroencephalogram 84
Elimination disorders 23
Emotional Blunting 30
Emotional incontinence 44
Uncopresis 23
Endocrine disorders 86
Endomorph 12
Enuresis 23
Epilepsy 10, 59, 95
Examination 7
Experiences of Alienation 45
Experiences of Influence 45
Expressive prosody 80

Factitious Disorder 58
First-Rank Symptoms of Schneider 39, 45
Flight of ideas 73
Fluent Aphasias 78

Fluoxetine 55, 56, 100, 101
Fluphenazine 40
Flurazeparn 103
Form 98
Fregoli's Syndrome 82
Freud 18

GABA 93
Gait 12
Gamma-aminobutyfic acid 93
Gegenhalten 29, 75, 91
Gender Identity Disorders 61, 62
Generalized Anxiety Disorder 23, 55
Generalized seizures 95
Gerstmann's syndrome 90, 92
Gesturing 80
Gilles de la Tourette's 22
Global aphasia 78
Graphesthesia 83, 92

Hallucinations 8, 39, 40, 43, 73
Hallucinogens 34, 35, 36
Haloperidol 22, 28, 40, 49, 55
Handedness 76
Harm avoidance 69
Hashish 36
Head Trauma Syndromes 94
Headaches 94
Heroin 32, 34, 37
Herpes Encephalitis 87
Histrionic 67
Histrionic personality disorder 68
HIV 35
Huntington's chorea 10, 12, 25
Hydrocephaly 8, 11
Hyperactivity 13
Hyperprolactinernia 99
Hypersexuality 61
Hypertensive crisis 101
Hypnotics 34
Hypoactivity 13
Hypochondriasis 58
Hypomania 49
Hysteria S7

ICD-9; 9
Ictal 96
Id 18
Ideomotor praxis 76
Idiokinetic dyspraxia 76, 77

Imipramine 56
Induced psychotic disorder 42
Inductive data 71
Inhalants 34, 36, 37
Insomnia 65, 66, 103
Intensity of affect 16
Interictal 96, 97
Intoxication 59
Irritable bowel syndrome 54

Jactacio nocturnus 66
Jamais vu 44
Jargon speech 11, 78

Kinesthetic praxis 76
Kleine-Levin Syndrome 61
Kluver-Bucy Syndrome 61

Lab Test 86
Language 9, 77
Late-Luteal Phase Syndrome 51
Learning Disorders 19
Left-right disorientation 92
Lethal catatonia 51
Lithium 14, 40, 48, 49, 101, 102
Lorazepam 29, 46, 103
LSD 35, 37, 46
Lysergic acid diethylamide (LSD) 35

Magnesium sulfate 33
Magnetic Resonance Imaging 85
Malingering 58
Mania 8, 93, 101, 108
Manic-depressive 47
Mannerisms 13
MAOI's 48, 54, 56, 100
Marijuana 35, 36, 37
Medroxyprogesterone 62
Melancholia 8, 9, 47, 48, 49, 108
Memory 72, 73, 81, 98
Mental Retardation 19
Mental status examination 71, 72
Meprobarnate 34
Methadone 32
Methylphenidate 21
Migraine headaches 94
Mini-Mental Status exam 74
Mitral valve prolapse 54
Monoamineoxidase Inhibitors 14, 48, 56, 100, 101
Mood 15, 72, 73, 98

Mood Disorders 8, 47
Motor Behavior 75
Motor Functions 74
Motor Impersistence 91
Motor Inertia, 75
Motor Sequencing 75
Multi-infarct dementia 27
Multiaxial System 7
Multiple Sclerosis 10
Mushrooms 37
Mutism 30

Narcissistic personality disorder 68
Narcolepsy 65
Neologisms 87
Neuroimaging 85
Neuroleptic Malignant Syndrome 46, 99
Neuroleptics 14, 15, 30, 39, 99
Neurologic Exam 74
Neuropsychiatry 71
Neuropsychological Testing 86
Neurosis 53
Neurosurgery 56
Neurotic depression 49
Neurotransmitter 93
Nicotine 34
Night terrors 65, 66
Nonfluent aphasias 77
Nonmelancholic Depression 48
Novelty seeking 69

Obsessional Syndromes 54
Obsessive-Compulsive Disorder 22, 54, 55, 70
Obsessive-Compulsive personality disorder 67, 69
Omega sign 47, 73
Oneiroid 95
Opiate addiction 35
Opiates 34, 37
Oppositional Defiant Disorder 22
Opthalmoplegia 33
Orbitomedial Syndrome 88
Organic mental disorders 47

Panic attack 53
Panic disorder 53, 56
Paranoid 67
Paranoid personality disorder 69
Paranoid type-Schizophrenia 42
Paraphasia 11, 87
Paraphilias 62

Paraphrenia 42
Parasomnias 65, 66
Parietal Lobe Syndrome 90
Parkinsonism 14
Passive-Aggressive 70
Pavor nocturnus 66
PCP 35, 36, 37, 46
Pernoline 21
Penicillamine 27
Penicillin 28
Perceptions 43
Perseveration 87, 91
Personality Disorders 67, 68, 69
Pervasive Developmental Disorders 22, 24
Petit mal seizure 84
Phencyclidine 35, 36, 37
Phenelzine 56, 100
Phenothiazines 14
Phentolamine 101
Phobias 54
Photosensitivity 99
PICA 22
Pick's Disease 27
PMS 51
Positron Emission Tomography 85
Post-Concussion Syndrome 94
Post-Traumatic Dementia 94
Post-Traumatic Stress Disorder 55
Post-Traumatic Thalamic Syndrome 94
Postictal 96
Postpartum Psychosis 45
Premature ejaculation 61, 62
Premenstrual Syndrome 51
Problem Solving 80
Prodromal 96
Prosody 80
Prosopagnosia 82
Prozac 55, 56, 100, 101
Pseudoseizures 97
Psilocybin 35, 46
Psychiatric Interview 71
Psychoanalytic Theory 18
Psychomotor activity 72
Psychopathology 10
Psychopharmacology 99
Psychosensory Symptoms 44
Psychosis 12, 36, 40, 45, 46, 97
Psychotic Depression 48
Psychotic Disorders 41

Rambling speech 8
Range of affect 16
Rapid-Cycling Pattern 52
Reactive Depression 48
Reasoning 80
Receptive prosody 80
Relatedness 16
Repetitive movements 55
Residual type 42
Rett's Disorder 24
Reward dependence 69
Right Hemisphere Syndrome 89
Ritalin® 21
Rumination disorder 22

Satiety 93
Schizoaffective disorder 39, 41, 42
Schizoid 67
Schizoid personality disorder 69
Schizophrenia 8, 11, 12, 30, 39, 40, 41, 42, 108
Schizophreniform Disorder 41, 42
Schizotypal 67
Schizotypal personality disorder 69
Seasonal Pattern 52
Secondary Depression 51
Sedation Threshold Test 49
Sedative Hypnotics 34, 37
Sedatives 104
Seizure Disorders 95
Selegiline 28
Self-help groups 32
Separation Anxiety 23
Serotonin 64, 93
Serotonin- selective reuptake inhibitors 55
Sexual Aversion Disorder 61
Sexual Dysfunction 61
Sexually Deviant Behavior 61
Shared Psychotic Disorder 41
Sleep Apnea 65
Sleep Disorders 65, 66
Social Phobia 22
Sodium amobarbital 29
Sodium bicarbonate 53
Sodium lactate 53
Soft neurologic signs 75
Somatic Anxiety 53
Somatization Disorder 57
Somatoform Disorders 57
Somatoform Pain disorder 58
Somnambulism 65

SPECT 85
Speech 9, 72, 77, 87, 92
Squeeze Technique 62
SSRI's 56
Stereognosis 83
Stereotypy 30
Steroids 37
Stimulant addiction 35
Stimulants 34
Stimulus-bound motor behavior 75
Stranger anxiety 23
Stupor 13, 29, 74
Subcortical Dementias 27
Substance Abuse Disorders 31
Substance-Induced Psychosis 41
Succinylecholine 107
Suicide 50
Superego 18
Syphilis 86

Tacrine 26
Tangential speech 11, 87
Tardive dyskinesia 13, 15, 40
Temazepam 103
Temporal Lobe Epilepsy 95, 96
Temporal Lobe Syndrome 89
Tension Headaches 94
Tetrahydrocannabinol 35, 36
Thalamic Aphasia 78, 79, 92
THC 35
Thiamine 33
Thiamine deficiency 33
Thinking 80
Thought Broadcasting 45
Thought Content 98
Thought Disorder 11, 30
Thought Processes 73
Thought Processing 72
Thyroid function tests 86
Tic Disorders 22
Tics 55
Tobacco 34
Tolerance 31, 36
Tourette's Syndrome 10, 22, 55
Transcortical motor aphasia 78
Transcortical sensory aphasia 78
Transsexualism 62
Transvestism 62
Tranylcypromine 100
Tri-cyclic antidepressants 14

Triazolam 103
Tricyclic antidepressants 54, 56
Tyramine 101

Undifferentiated type-Schizophrenia 42

Vaginismus 61, 62
Valproic acid 44, 102, 103
VDRL 86
Veraguth's folds 47
Verbigeration 87
Visceral hallucinations 44
Visual memory 81
Visual-Spatial function 82
Vitamin B12 deficiency 25
Vitamins 27, 33
Volition 16

Waxy flexibility 30
Wernicke's Aphasia 77, 78, 79
Wernicke's Encephalopathy 86
Wernicke-Korsakoff's Syndrome 32, 33
Wilson's disease 27
Withdrawal Syndrome 32, 36
Word Approximations 11, 87

Additional References

American Psychiatric Association: Diagnostic and Statistical Manual of Mental Disorders, Fourth Edition, Washington, DC, APA, 1994.

Golbin, Alexander, M.D., Ph.D., The World of Children's Sleep, Chicago, IL, Michaelis Medical Publishing Corp., 1995.

Kaplan, H.I., Sadock, B.J., Kaplan & Sadock's Synopsis of Psychiatry, Baltimore, MD, Williams & Wilkins, 1994.

Kaplan, H.I., Sadock, B.J., Comprehensive Textbook of Psychiatry, Baltimore, MD, Williams & Wilkins, 1989.

Merck Sharp & Dohme Research Labs., The Merck Manual of Diagnosis and Therapy, Sixteenth edition, Rahway, NJ, Merck, 1994.

NOTES

NOTES

NOTES

NOTES

NOTES

NOTES

NOTES

ISBN 0-07-038219-0

LINARDAKIS:
PSYCHIATRY